SunLight Chair Yoga: yoga for everyone!

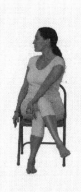

SunLight Chair Yoga: yoga for everyone!

Copyright © 2014 Stacie Dooreck

Not all of the yoga postures and exercises in this book are suitable for everyone. Consult your physician or medical provider for concerns prior to doing these exercises. The instructions and suggestions in this book are in no way intended as a substitute for medical counseling.

SunLight Yoga Publishers

ISBN-10: 0991625021
ISBN-13: 978-0-9916250-2-4
BISAC: Health & Fitness / Yoga
Second Edition (Black and White) Jan 2014

Printed in the United States of America

"Expand. Evolve. Grow. Forget not the goal. Awake. Achieve the goal." Swami Sivananda

REVIEWS

"Sunlight Chair Yoga shines new, beautiful, creative energy on a subject whose time has finally come...Chair Yoga! Artfully modified yoga moves in a chair. Stretches, breathing and relaxation for men and women of all ages. Lovely color photos, clear directions sharing the benefits of Yoga for every - BODY. Thank you Stacie Dooreck! -Lilias Folan, Swami Kavitananda, PBS Lilias! Yoga and You Author Lilias! Yoga - Your Guide to Enhancing Body, Mind and Spirit Midlife and Beyond www.liliasyoga.com

"Good stuff! We use her tips here in the office." Marin Magazine editor Mimi Towle

"The book is so beautifully and professionally printed, with lots of photographs. It was just what I was looking for. Thank you for making this available to us, Stacie...It looks like dozens of ideas, just as you promised!" Jane

"Just got the book today. Absorbed it in a day. Loved it. Liked the section about yoga works at work. Thank you!" Gail, Chair Yoga Instructor; Texas

'I'm enjoying it already. So I am happy I ordered it." Yoga Instructor, Netherlands

"For those of you who sit in a chair all day and need some simple tools to stretch, I highly recommend Stacie's new book, Sunlight Chair Yoga: Yoga for Everyone!" Ingrid, LA Chair Yoga Teacher

DEDICATION

To my father who brought yoga into my life and continues to keep it in his.

And to my mom, who supported our vegetarian diet and my life work as a yoga instructor.

ACKNOWLEDGMENTS

To all of my "chair yoga" students, who were also my teachers as I wrote my first SunLight Chair Yoga teacher training manual and this SunLight Chair Yoga book.

To all yoga masters including: Swami Sivananda, Krishnamacharya, Swami Vishnu Devananda, Swami Sachidnananda, BKS Iyengar, Yogi Bhajan and Pattabhi Jois. Their teachings are timeless yet perfect for the modern age.

To the yoga teachers in the USA who have influenced and inspired my own yoga practice and teachings including Lilias Folan, Dharma Mittra and Gurmukh Kaur Khalsa.

I am very grateful to the lineages of yoga that I have learned from and experienced including: Sivananda Yoga for the foundation of hatha yoga (postures, pranayama, relaxation and meditation), Integral Yoga for Gentle Yoga adaption ideas and Kundalini Yoga for it's tools to increase and contain the *prana* (vital life force) for healing and well being.

Wahe Guru! Victory to the True Teacher within!

QUOTES FROM THE MASTERS

"The human body is a temple. Keep it strong and supple. Treat it gently." Swami Sachidananda

"Health is wealth. Peace of mind is happiness. Yoga shows the way." Swami Vishnudevananda

"If you can breathe, you can do yoga."
Krishnamacharya

"Yoga teaches us to cure what need not be endured and endure what cannot be cured." BKS Iyengar

"The highest point of yesterday should be the lowest point of today." BKS Iyengar

"The Nature of the Absolute is Peace: Absolute Peace, Perfect Peace, Unutterable Peace."
Swami Sivananda

"Serve, love, give, purify,
meditate, realize.

Be good, do good, be kind,
be compassionate.

Inquire 'who am I'
know the Self and be free...

Concentrate, meditate,
attain Self-realization."

–Swami Sivananda

TABLE OF CONTENTS

CHAIR YOGA

When there are physical, energetic, time or other "limitations," the benefits of yoga can still be experienced. When yoga is done in ways that are comfortable, safe and within range of one's current capabilities, the healing, balancing and transformative effects of yoga can occur. Often when we are sick, injured, fatigued or busy at the office, the last thing we think we can do is yoga. But when we modify it to meet our current needs instead of avoiding the practice altogether, yoga can bring peace of mind, inner and outer strength, flexibility (mental and physical), stress relief, vitality, energy, overall well-being, balance and joy. Yoga is for everyone!

What is yoga?

The word yoga comes form the Sanskrit language, meaning to "yoke" or "join". The "yoking" or "joining" or connecting of the individual self (soul) with the Universal or Cosmic Self (Soul) is Yoga. It is the connection of our individual selves to all that exists in the universe that is Yoga, including every human being, animal, tree and atom. On a simple level, yoga connects the body, mind and Spirit, often using the breath as one tool to connect those parts. Yoga also unifies, balances and harmonizes our physical, emotional, mental and spiritual selves.

Yoga is a science of sorts. You must not believe any claims until you try it for yourself and experience its benefits firsthand. The benefits are as infinite as our true selves. With practice, anyone can experience this.

Patanjali, a sage of India consolidated yoga into stages or limbs (*ashtanga* in Sanskrit) known as the 8 limbs of yoga. These include ethics such as nonviolence or *ahimsa* in Sanskrit, truthfulness *(satya)* and study of the true Self *(svadhyaya)*. After the ethical standards of what to do and not do for living a life with true integrity Patanjali notes the third limb as yoga *asana* or posture. The Chair Yoga postures in this book are adaptions using chairs for support of traditional or more modern variations of yoga postures and exercises.

Following yoga *asana* is pranayama, or yogic breathing practices, for balancing and/or increasing the *prana* (vital life force). Then comes *pratyahara,* which is turning the senses inward. After that is *dharana* or concentration and *dhyana* (meditation) leading up to the final stage of *Samadhi*, which is the realization that all is One and is said to be a state of pure ecstasy. Although these stages can go in the above order, they may also overlap and vary in sequence. You can also practice several of these at once. For example, taking a slow, deep breath during the yoga posture while concentrating deeply can be considered doing an *asana* (yoga posture) *pranayama* (yogic breathing exercises) and *dharana* (concentration) simultaneously. Perhaps you can also ease into a state of *dhyana* (meditation) during the practice. Each time you practice yoga is an opportunity to be present and observe yourself without judgment. And of course, don't forget to enjoy the journey!

"The human body is a temple. Keep it strong and supple. Treat it gently. The codes of living, *Yama* and *Niyama*, are the first two limbs of the eight branches of Yoga. The third is asana--Yoga postures that purify the physical body. Never ignore the body since it is the most important instrument. Whatever you do, you need a body. That's why the ancient Yoga teachings always emphasized taking good care of the body. In almost all the great religious traditions this is indirectly said, but not as openly or with such emphasis as in Yoga. To purify the body we practice the disciplines of Hatha Yoga, the asanas or--postures and *pranayama*--the breathing techniques, which take care of the health of the physical body. This carries over into diet too. Avoid anything that contains toxins or that unnecessarily stimulates your body; try to eliminate alcohol and tobacco. Without purity of the body it's very difficult to purify the mind." –Swami Sachidananda

What is Chair Yoga?

Chair Yoga is simply yoga done in a chair or wheelchair, (seated or standing), using the chair as a prop for support and stability. The main difference between yoga and chair yoga is that while the yoga postures are sometimes adapted from traditional postures, we are using the chair as support as well. Being creative makes yoga accessible for all.

SunLight Chair Yoga's suggested yoga session includes centering, yoga warm-ups, yoga exercises and postures, concentration and breathing exercises, yogic relaxation, meditation and chanting. Although any one of these elements alone can bring great benefit, practicing all of them will give the maximum results for a healthy body, peaceful mind and joyful Spirit.

For Chair Yoga specifically, even if you have little or no physical movement ability, there are numerous benefits. This includes the calming of the nervous system and mind (from yogic breathing exercises and mantras), the social benefits if practiced with others, as well as giving one a purpose, challenge and sense of accomplishment after practicing and doing something productive. Yoga is a discipline with great rewards.

What are the benefits of Chair Yoga?

Doing yoga in chairs gives the same benefits as any other yoga practice does, relative to the practitioner's abilities and capabilities. Just like all yoga (when applied holistically and safely), Chair Yoga can give you more flexibility (in body and mind), physical and mental strength, increased energy and vitality, improved memory and clarity and better concentration. It can improve overall feelings of health, vitality and peace. Just taking time for yourself a few minutes a day to benefit your well being can be an accomplishment in itself.

Who can do Chair Yoga?

Everyone can do yoga! Chair Yoga is a safe and effective way to practice yoga at any age and level of health, ability or mobility. This includes doing yoga:

- At work (at your desk)
- On airplanes
- With limited mobility
- For a gentle yoga practice
- With an acute or chronic illness
- Pre- and post surgery
- While healing from an injury
- In a wheelchair
- While pregnant
- In a hospital or rehab center
- In an assisted living home
- With a support group
- While healing from posttraumatic stress

Options are available for certain yoga postures to sit or stand (using the chair back as support if needed). If you are unable to do the standing version, you can do the upper body movements while seated, or modify as you need to so that you are comfortable, safe and at ease. For those with limited physical mobility or energy limitations, the breathing exercises, mental concentration, and relaxation alone are enough without the physical exercises, so that truly: yoga is for everyone!

What do you wear for Chair Yoga?

Anything you want! This can make Chair Yoga more accessible to some than a yoga class at a studio or health club that may require a change of clothes and more time to prepare.

At work, you can do Chair Yoga in business attire and with shoes on. In general, however, it is advised to wear comfortable clothes you can stretch in, but it is not necessary. Yoga can be done in shoes, socks or bare feet. If the standing postures are practiced, please note that bare feet are preferable to avoid slipping. Keep in mind that yoga is not just about the physical exercises and postures alone, but it includes breathing and meditation. That can be done anywhere and anytime, starting with a slow, deep breath.

When do you do Chair Yoga?

You can do Chair Yoga anytime and anywhere. Since the yoga practice includes breathing exercises, meditation and concentration exercises, you can even do it in environments where you do not want to do active yoga postures and exercises. In fact, no one will even know you are practicing yoga except for the fact that they will see how much more calm, refreshed and content you may seem afterwards. Even one minute a day helps, so try it whenever and wherever you can.

If you want to establish a daily practice, which is recommended for progress, easing pain and discomfort, general wellness maintenance and even prevention of possible future aches and pains, consistent daily practice will produce the best results. However, do not be discouraged if your schedule, energy level or health prevents you from practicing Chair Yoga as much as you would like or intend to. Just start where you are with one minute a day and progress from there as you are able.

If you create the same time of day to practice, that will allow the mind and body to create a habit, so that less motivation and effort is required as time goes on to practice. That is because you will want to practice out of the experience of feeling better day to day when you do. However, be gentle with yourself if you miss a day and start again when you are able.

What Type of Chair do you use?

It is best to use a chair that is not on wheels, if it is available for more stability. However at work or in an office or hospital setting, for example, if that is all you have available just be mindful to not slip or put the chair against a wall if able. This book uses the word "chair" which can be interchanged with how do yoga in a wheelchair, on a couch, on an airplane seat or in other settings when adapting traditional yoga postures is appropriate.

An example of a sturdy metal chair that is useful for Chair Yoga is displayed in the photos on the following page. The chairs in the yoga posture demonstrations in this book have an open back and are commonly found at yoga studios. However, some chairs have arms on the sides, which can be useful for spinal twists (to rest the arms). Try to get creative and adapt the ideas for doing yoga in a chair as best you can based on the space and chairs that you have available.

Chair Photos

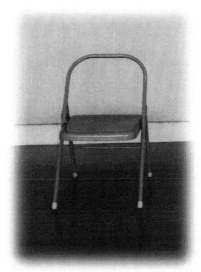

Chair Without a Back

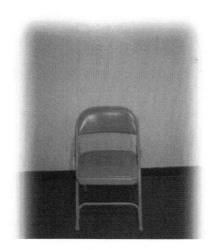

Chair With a Back

SunLight Chair Yoga Practice Includes:

For the best results, include the following elements in your yoga practice. For shorter practices (at work or on planes) even one part of this or practicing for just one minute is still useful. The acronym 'CHAIR' is one way to remember:

Centering (breathing or meditation)

Heating (warm-ups)

Asanas (postures) or yoga exercises

Inversions or Integration (meditation)

Relaxation (recharge, rest & renew)

CENTERING

Easy Pose (*Sukhasana*)

Sit tall in your chair with the feet hip-width apart and your heels under the knees (if able). See that the toes point forward. If comfortable, sit away from the chair back and lift from the base of your spine through the "crown" of the head (middle center of the top of the skull). Allow the hands to rest on the thighs with the palms up or down or place the hands together in front of the sternum (chest bone). The prayer pose is called *Anjali Mudra,* which is a devotional hand posture called a *mudra*, in Sanskrit.

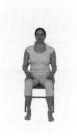 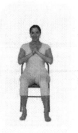

Easy Pose   *With Palms in Prayer*

In Easy Pose take a few slow, deep breaths to get centered. Bring your awareness to the present moment, feeling your body and the breath as it connects to the body. Inhale to lift the spine and exhale to relax into your posture. Relax your shoulders, your jaw and your eyes. Go through your body to check for areas that are holding on to extra physical tension (called a "body scan"). After observing your body and breath, still sitting tall but relaxed, begin to notice any thoughts as they arise, not accessing or judging any thoughts. Just be a silent witness.

TUNING IN WITH MANTRAS

If you resonate to do so, you can tune in with a simple Sanskrit mantra. A mantra is a repetitive sound or mind projection of a sound current that the mind can associate with a positive, calming or uplifting image or vibration. The yogic sound currents allow the mind to shift from the busyness and business of the day to the inner world where peace and tranquility reside.

In Easy Pose, allow the hands to rest on the thighs with the palms up or down or place the hands together in front of the sternum (chest bone). The prayer pose is called *Anjali Mudra,* which is a devotional hand posture called a *mudra*, in Sanskrit.

Inhale deeply. As you exhale, chant AUM (OM) 3x silently or out loud. Allow the sound to wash away all of your worries and thoughts of the world. Chant 'shanti' as listed below which means peace in Sanskrit. Tune in to the inner peace deep inside.

AUM (OM) 3X

Aum Shanti Shanti Shanti
Aum Peace Peace Peace

ॐ शान्तिः शान्तिः शान्तिः

YOGA EXERCISES AND POSTURES

Yoga is not the same as exercise as you may know it. The yoga exercises are to be done in a way that is a gentle, comfortable and relaxing practice for your body and mind. Even if the muscles of the body are working hard, it is more beneficial and recommended to only go as far as you are comfortable and to take breaks as needed. Especially if you are healing from an injury or dealing with certain aches and pains, make sure the yoga is easing them, or at least not aggravating any preexisting condition or injury.

Yoga postures, called "asanas" in Sanskrit, are defined by the Yoga Sutras of Patanjali as a steady, but comfortable, seat for meditation. It also says "posture is mastered by releasing tension and meditating on the Infinite or Unlimited." (Yoga Sutra 2.47) Based on that, for the maximum benefit, make sure that the body is comfortable in all postures and exercises. Some of the movements in this book are modified from the classic yoga postures and others are created for the modern age.

Please consult your doctor or medical provider for any questions or concerns for specific illnesses, ailments or injuries or any other health concerns, especially if you are not sure what you can and cannot do. For prenatal modifications, only do what is comfortable. Consult your doctor about any additional questions. All postures in this book are safe for all trimesters, except spinal twists. If you are pregnant you can twist from the upper body only (the shoulders, neck and head).

Suggested Yoga Practice Sequencing:

Each time you practice, if time allows, try to include at least one of the following exercises and/or postures on the following page from each section in your practice session. You can make this a 10-minute, 20-minute, 30-minute or 60-minute "hOMe" practice, for example, or for longer if time allows. Be practical and set realistic goals for a daily practice that works with your lifestyle and energy levels. Even one minute a day will help your well being and you can increase the time from there, as you feel inspired.

10-minute practice example:

1-min Meditation and Centering

3-min Warm Ups (Ex: Ankle and Wrist Rotations)

4-min Sun Salutations (Standing or Seated)

1-min Spinal Twist

1-min Relax and/or Breathing Exercises

30-minute practice example:

2-min Meditation and Centering

3-min Warm Ups

(Ex: Shoulder, Knee Swings and Spinal Warm Ups)

5-min Sun Salutations (Standing or Seated)

10-min Postures (Ex: Triangle Pose, Balance Poses)

5-min Relaxation Pose

5-min Breathing Exercises

Suggested Yoga Practice Sequencing Contents:

- **Warm Ups**
- **Sun Salutes**
- **Forward Bends**
- **Side Bends**
- **Spinal Twists**
- **Backbends**
- **Balance Poses**
- **Inversions**
- **Relaxation**
- **Breathing Exercises**
- **Meditation**
- **Mantras**

WARM UPS

Hand and Finger Stretch

Make fists, then extend/stretch your fingers/hands.
Repeat 5x.

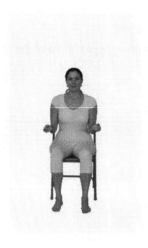
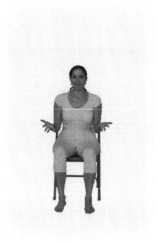

Inhale, Squeeze   *Exhale, Stretch*

Benefits: Stretches and strengthens the hands. This is a useful break to take from long hours at a computer.

Infinity Wrist Movements

Make figure eights in the air (infinity symbol) with your hands. Switch directions. Make bigger movements for upper body and shoulder warm-ups, moving the arms.

Benefits: Warms up and brings mobility to the wrist, shoulder and elbow joints. Increases circulation in the wrists.

Wrist Rotations

Rotate your hands around your wrists 3 to 6x. Make circles in the air with your fingers. Make circles with closed fists or open hands. Reverse directions and repeat 3 to 6x.

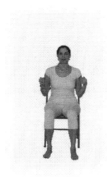
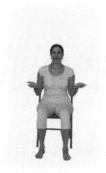

Fingers Inwards   *Circling Away*

Benefits: Improves the range of motion in the wrist joints. Increases the ability to adapt to changes when getting up from chairs, out of bed, etc. Eases wrist strain from computer use.

Point and Flex Foot Movements

Lift both feet a few inches off the ground. Slowly point your toes towards the floor then gently pull your toes back towards you 5 to 8x.

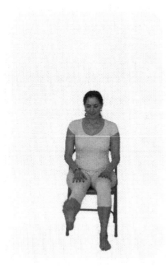 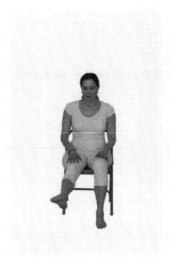

Toes Pointed   *Foot Flexed*

Benefits: Improves the range of motion in the ankles. This can be done at your desk, on airplanes, on the couch or in a wheelchair.

Toe and Heel Lifts and Rolls

Seated Lifts: Inhale as you lift your heels up. Exhale as you lower the heels down. You can lift each heel, one at a time, alternating or both together at the same time. Repeat 5x. Then do the same exercise lifting the toes, alternating sides or with both feet together.

Standing: Hold on to the chair back for support and repeat the exercise 5x using the same steps described above.

Rolls: Roll the weight back and forth between the toes and the heels. Repeat 5 to 8x.

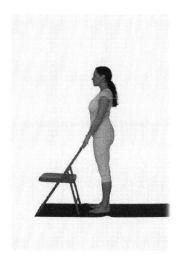

Standing: Center Position

Benefits: Strengthens the lower leg (calf and shin) and keeps the feet active and mobile. The standing version helps create balance and brings awareness to the base of the foot, which can prevent falls. It also gives the feet and lower legs the actions of moving with support from a chair.

Ankle Rotations

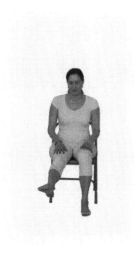

Ankle Rotations

Seated: Rotate your feet around your ankles 3 to 6x. Make circles in the air with your big toes. Make circles with one foot at a time or with both feet together at the same time. Reverse directions and repeat 3 to 6x. Then rotate one foot clockwise and the other counterclockwise. Switch sides.

Standing: Stand behind a chair with the toes pointing forward and the feet hip width apart. Place the hands on the top of the chair back for support. Lift one heel (or foot) and rotate one foot around the ankle 3 to 6x. Make circles in the air with your big toe. Reverse directions and then switch sides.

Benefits: Improves the range of motion and balance in the feet and ankles and the ability to adapt to changes when getting up from chairs, out of bed, etc. This can help to increase the circulation in the legs and feet. It helps to ease the joints on flights or during long meetings or days at your desk. The standing version strengthens the legs and increases balance.

Prayer Pose (*Anjali Mudra*)

Place your hands together in prayer position in front of the heart area. Place your thumbs on your sternum. Relax your shoulders.

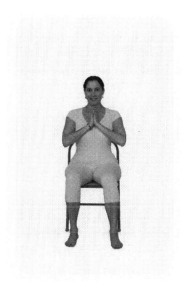

Prayer Pose

Benefits: This brings the attention to the heart area and allows the mind to focus inward. This is also a symbol and reminder of our devotional nature and perhaps reminds us to take a moment to feel grateful and faithful.

Prayer Pose Exercises

1- *Rotations:* Bring your palms into Prayer Pose. (See photo) Rotate your fingers towards your heart, then towards the floor in front of you. Repeat 5x.

2- *Push Hands*: In Prayer Pose, push your hands from side to side. Feel resistance from the hand you are pushing into.

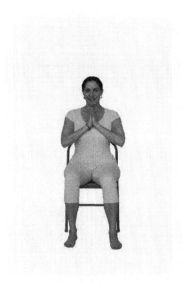

Prayer Pose

Benefits: Warms up and loosens the wrists (Rotations) upper back and shoulders (Push Hands). This eases strain from computer use or repetitive movements and for those sitting long hours at a desk.

Sacred Circles

From Prayer Pose, inhale and stretch the hands up, keeping your palms together. Exhale as you separate the hands away from each other and draw a big circle around you. Inhale as you join the palms back to Prayer Pose at the navel center and stretch up again. Repeat 5 to 8x.

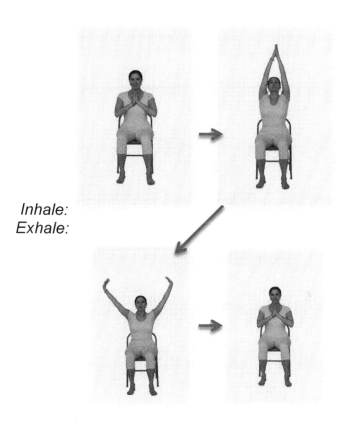

Inhale:
Exhale:

Benefits: Warms up and loosens the upper back and shoulders, increases circulation and stretches the hands and arms (good for computer use and for those sitting long hours at a desk). Imagine you're pushing away any negativity or energies you don't need. Also, this coordinates the breath with the body for mental calming and soothing of the nervous system. This can be done before any yoga practice or by itself as a one-minute stretch break while at work.

Reverse Prayer Pose and Sacred Circles

Reverse Namaste: Bring your hands behind the back. Hold on to your elbows or wrists or fingers. If you are able, place the palms in prayer position behind your back. Take 3 to 5 slow, deep breaths as you feel the upper back and shoulders opening.

Reverse Sacred Circles: Inhale and stretch the hands up with the palms facing skyward. Exhale as you bring the palms to Prayer Pose overhead and then to the sternum (chest bone). Repeat 5-8x. *(See photos)*

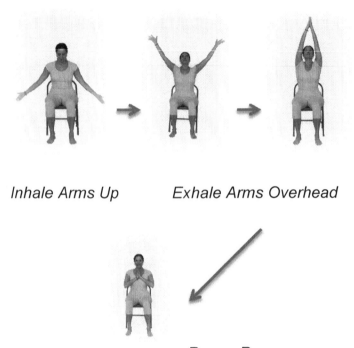

Inhale Arms Up   *Exhale Arms Overhead*

Prayer Pose

Benefits: Warms up and loosens the upper back and shoulders, increases circulation and stretches the hands and arms (good for computer use and for those sitting long hours at a desk), and coordinates the breath with the body for mental calming. You can imagine you are gathering energy *(prana)* with your hands.

Seated Cat Cow Poses

From Seated Mountain Pose, inhale as you lift the heart into an upper back bend, sliding the hands towards the hips. Exhale as you round at the navel point (belly button) and round the upper back, reaching the hands towards the knees. Or keep the arms straight with the hands above the knees the whole time. Keep the head centered. Repeat 4 to 8x. Feel the spine move like a wave in a meditative, rhythmic motion.

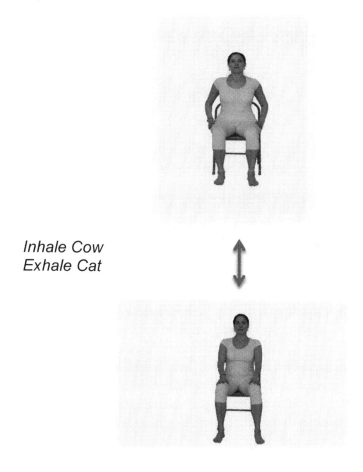

Inhale Cow
Exhale Cat

Benefits: Warms up the spine, eases back tension and increases energy.

"Sufi Grind" (from Kundalini Yoga)

Sit tall in your chair with the feet hip width apart. Inhale as you lean slightly back and to the right. Then exhale as you lean forward and to the left. Continue moving the spine in a circular direction, keeping the head upright. Repeat 5x: inhale as you lean back and exhale as you lean forward. Reverse direction.

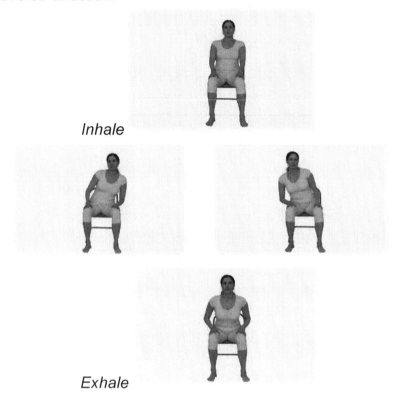

Inhale

Exhale

Benefits: Warms up the spine, hips and back, eases back tension, coordinates the breath with the body and mind and increases energy.

Shoulder Shrugs

Inhale and shrug the shoulders up to the ears. Exhale as you drop the shoulders down, away from the ears. Imagine that you are releasing all your tensions and worries with each exhalation. Repeat 3 to 6x.

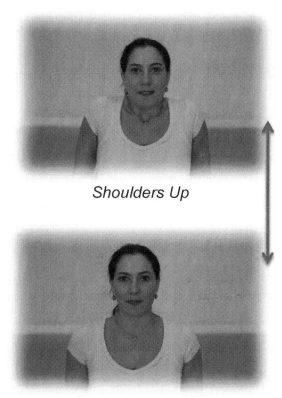

Shoulders Up

Shoulders Down

Benefits: Eases neck and shoulder tensions. Reminds the shoulders and upper back muscles to relax while on the computer or from general stress. This is helpful to remind the neck and shoulders to relax on airplanes or on long road trips.

Shoulder Rolls and Movements

1- Circle the shoulders forward 5 to 10x. Reverse direction. Move with your breath. For example, inhale when the shoulders are up and exhale when they are down.

2- Bring the hands to shoulders and make circles with your elbows: small circles at first and then bigger circles. Reverse direction, 5 to 10x each. Move with your breath. For example, inhale when the elbows are up and exhale when the elbows are down.

3- Inhale as you move the elbows away from each other towards the wall behind you. Exhale as you move the elbows towards each other or touching. Repeat 3 to 5x.

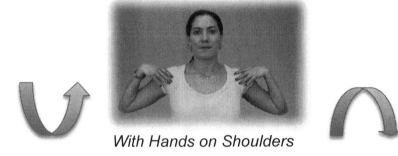

With Hands on Shoulders

Benefits: Eases shoulder and neck tension, increases mobility to the shoulder joint and rotator cuff, increases circulation, expands and relaxes the upper chest and tones the upper arms. This can be done at work or on an airplane for quick shoulder relief from muscular or mental tension.

Precautions: For shoulder pain, make smaller circles.

Shoulder Mobility Exercise

Props needed: Yoga belt (or strap, scarf or towel)

Place one side of the belt in each hand between the thumb and index (first) finger. Separate the hands wider than shoulder-width apart. (See photo below) Inhale as you lift the belt overhead or as far as comfortable (shoulder height if needed). Exhale as you lower the belt towards the thighs or touch the thighs. Add neck exercises by looking up as you lift the belt overhead, and looking down as you lower it. Repeat 5 to 8x.

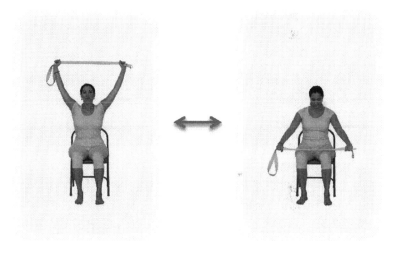

Inhale the Arms Up   *Exhale the Arms Down*

Benefits: Increases shoulder mobility and range of motion. Expands the chest and upper body. Helps you feel like you have more room to breathe (mentally and physically).

Neck Stretch

Inhale as sit tall and center your head. Exhale as you lower your right ear to your right shoulder. Keep the shoulders relaxed. Switch sides. Repeat 5x in each direction.

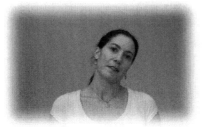

Neck Stretch

Benefits: Eases neck tension and stretches the sides of the neck.

Neck Turns

Turn your head side to side. Inhale as you bring your head to the center. Exhale as you turn your head to one side, looking over your shoulder as far as you are comfortable. Relax the shoulders and jaw as you sit tall. Move your eyes to each side with the neck movements. Switch sides. Repeat 5x in each direction.

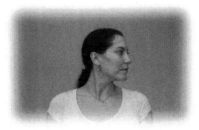

Neck Turns

Benefits: Eases neck tension and brings mobility to the neck. Relieves computer-related neck tension or general dullness from lack of movement.

Half Neck Circles

Rotate the neck in half circles. Inhale as you lift one ear to your shoulder. Exhale as you bring the chin down towards your chest bone. Switch sides. Repeat 5x in each direction.

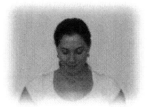

Head Down

Benefits: Eases neck tension and brings mobility to the neck. This is useful on long flights or after computer use.

Full Neck Circles

Center the head over the spine. Draw 5 circles in the air with your nose. Inhale when the nose (chin) is up, and exhale when the nose (chin) comes down. Reverse directions.

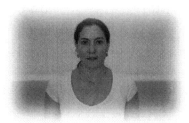

Head Centered

Benefits: Eases neck tension and increases neck mobility.

Precautions: For neck pain, move the *eyes only*.

Alternate Leg Raises

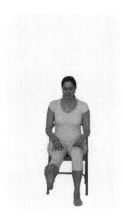

Inhale as you lift one foot/leg up (keep your thigh on the chair for support). Exhale as you lower. Switch legs. Repeat 5x on each side or as you are comfortable. Keep the back relaxed yet sitting tall.

Alternate Leg Raises

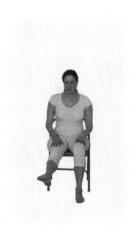

Point and Flex

Point and Flex Variation: Inhale as you point the toes and raise the lower leg. Exhale as you and flex the foot and lower the leg. Repeat 3 to 5x. Switch sides. Reverse by flexing the foot as you inhale and lift, and pointing the toes as you exhale and lower. Repeat 5x. Switch sides.

Benefits: Strengthens the quadriceps (muscles on the front of the thigh), helps the knee joint and stretches the legs. It brings circulation and energy to the legs and feet.

Arm Swings

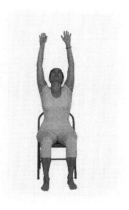

Inhale as you lift one arm up. Exhale as you swing the arm down, lowering the arm next to the side of the chair. Switch sides. Repeat 5x. Then swing both arms together 5x.

Arm Swings

Benefits: Improves shoulder mobility and the range of motion in the shoulder joints.

Leg Swings

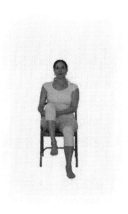

Place the hands under one knee and swing the foot back and forth. Switch sides. You can also keep the thigh on the chair base for support.

Leg Swings

Benefits: Improves mobility and range of motion in the knee joints.

Knee Circles

From Seated Lunge Pose (p. 44), make circles in the air with your knee. Repeat 5x. Reverse direction. Switch legs. Keep the spine tall. Relax the shoulders and jaw. The breathing is slow and deep. You can inhale as the knee is at the top of the circle, and exhale as the knee reaches the bottom of the circle.

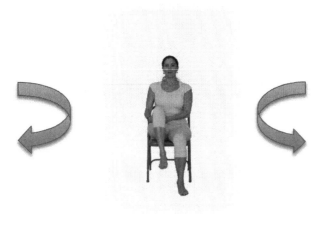

Knee Circles

Benefit: Increases knee mobility and can ease knee, hip and low back pain. Strengthens the back muscles (as all postures do) by keeping the spine tall.

Extended Hand to Foot Pose *(Hasta Padasana)*

Hold the leg that is stretched in the air under the thigh, or rest it on the chair base.

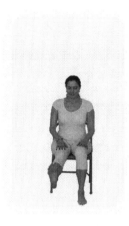

Leg On Chair Base

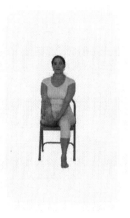

Holding the Leg

With Props: Place a belt or strap under the right foot. Inhale as you lift the right foot and as you extend the leg. Hold the belt with two hands, keeping the shoulders relaxed and the hands under the shoulders. Hold for 1-5 slow, deep breaths. Switch sides.

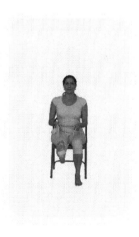

With a Belt

Benefits: Stretches the hamstrings, legs and calves.

Seated Extended Hand to Big Toe Pose
(Utthita Hasta Padangusthasana)

Props needed: Yoga belt (or strap, scarf or towel)

Place a belt around the right foot. Step on the belt as the foot is on the floor if needed. Keep the belt around the right foot (or hold your right big toe with your right index finger if comfortable). Hold one side of the belt in each hand. Pull against the belt to sit tall and stretch the leg. Keep the shoulders relaxed. Take 2 to 4 deep, slow, deep, rhythmic breaths. Switch sides.

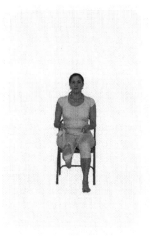

With A Belt

Benefits: Stretches the hamstrings, legs and calves.

Seated Extended Hand to Big Toe Pose Variation
(Utthita Hasta Padangusthasana)

Props needed: Yoga belt (or strap, scarf or towel)

From Extended Hand to Foot Pose (see photo on the previous page), keep the belt around the right foot (or hold your right big toe if comfortable). Take both sides of the belt into the right hand. Inhale as you sit tall and lift the left arm up. Exhale as you take your right foot out to the right. Then reach your left hand out to the left (while you stretch the right foot to the right at the same time). Look past the left fingertips as you keep the eyes relaxed. Keep the shoulders relaxed and the spine tall. Make sure that there is no strain. Take 2 to 4 deep, slow breaths. Switch sides.

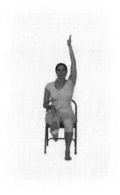

Left Arm Up

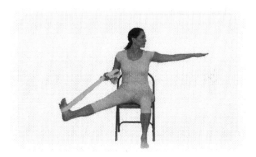

Seated Arm and Leg Balance

Benefits: Stretches the hamstrings and arm, coordinates the right and left sides of the brain and body and helps improves balance, focus and confidence.

Double Leg Raises

Sitting tall, with the hands on the sides of the chair base, chair arms or thighs, inhale as you lift both feet up (keep your thigh on the chair for support). Exhale as you lower. Repeat 5x. Keep the back relaxed yet sitting tall and away from the chair back.

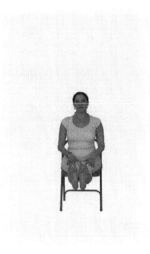

Double Leg Raises

Benefits: Strengthens the quadriceps (front thigh muscles), helps the knee joint and stretches the legs.

Staff Pose *(Dandasana)*

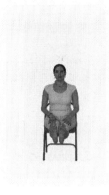

Inhale as stretch your legs out and up. Keep the thighs on the chair base for support. Hold the legs out as you take 2 to 4 slow, deep breaths. Feel the spine reaching towards the sky as the legs stretch away from the navel point (belly button area).

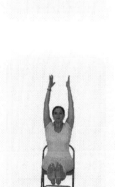

For a more active pose, reach the arms as well. Feel the arms and spine reaching towards the sky as the legs stretch away from the navel point.

Arms Up

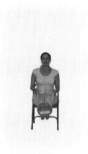

For more support, wrap a yoga belt (or towel) around your feet as in the photo on the left. Hold onto the belt with your hands. As you inhale pulll against the belt to sit tall, keeping the shoulders relaxed.

With a Belt

Benefits: Strengthens the back and quadriceps, and stretches the legs and arms. This also strengthens the muscles on the upper thigh, which supports the knee joint.

Staff Pose with Props *(Dandasana)*

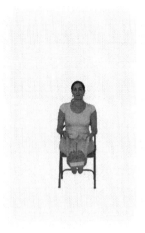

Place the belt under the toes. Hold one hand to each side of the belt. Inhale as you lift the legs. Keep the shoulders relaxed and the hands in line with your shoulders. Sit tall. Feel your body's strength.

With a Belt

Place the feet on top of a second chair in front of you for support. Relax the hands on the thighs or stretch the arms up overhead. Reach up with the fingertips and lengthen the spine as you stretch the heels away from the navel point (belly button).

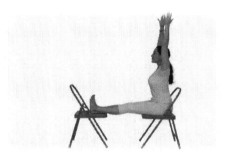

With Two Chairs

Benefits: Strengthens the back and muscles on the thighs (quadriceps) and stretches the legs and arms.

Upward Hand Pose *(Urdhva Hastasana)*

Stretch the arms up overhead. Hold and breath for 1 to 5 slow, deep breathes.

Single Arm Raises: Inhale as you lift one arm up overhead, as high as is comfortable for you. Exhale as you lower. Alternate arms. You can lower the arm to the side of the chair or to your lap. Repeat 5x on each side.

Double Arm Raises

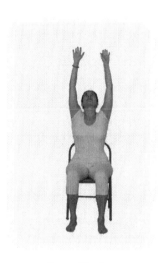

Arm Raises

Inhale as you lift both arms up overhead, as high as comfortable. Look up as you lift the arms to combine this with a neck movement. Exhale when you come down to lower the arms (and bring the head back to center if you were looking up). You can lower the arms to the side of the chair or to your lap. Repeat 5x.

Benefits: Increases circulation and coordination. It also strengthens the arms, mind-body connection and breath awareness. Brings mobility to the shoulder joints and neck (if you add the head movements).

Precautions: For neck pain, keep the head centered and look up with the eyes only. For shoulder injuries bring the arms up to shoulder height or as far as comfortable.

Arm and Leg Raises

Inhale as you lift your right arm up. At the same time extend your right leg out. Exhale to lower. Switch sides. Repeat 5x, alternating sides. (See photo below) Extend the arm and leg away from your navel point. Sit tall and keep your back and shoulders relaxed.

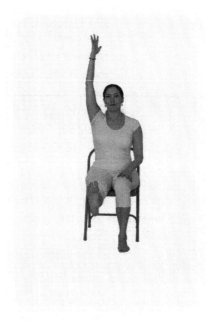

Arm and Leg Raises

Benefits: Improves leg and arm mobility, circulation, strength and coordination. This can energize sluggish or tired hands, arms, feet and legs and vitalize the body.

Alternating Arm and Leg Lifts

Inhale as you lift your right arm up, and extend the left leg out. Exhale as you lower the arm and leg. Switch sides and repeat 3 to 6x.

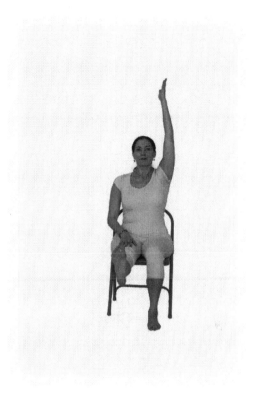

Alternating Arm and Leg Lifts

Benefits: Improves and increases coordination of the body and right and left sides of the brain, circulation, arm and leg mobility, range of motion in the shoulder and knee joints, and increases leg and arm strength.

Seated Mountain Pose *(Tadasana)*

Sit tall in your chair with the feet hip-width apart and your heels under your knees. See that the toes point forward. If comfortable, sit away from the chair back, and lift from the base of your spine through the "crown" of the head (middle center of the top of the skull). Allow the hands to rest on the thighs with the palms down. Feel your feet root into the earth like a mountain and the crown of the head reach towards the sky like a mountaintop.

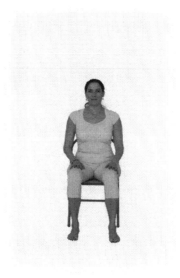

Mountain Pose

Benefits: Increases concentration, and stability, and gives the mind time to pause and get centered. Feeling the feet on the ground (earth) helps balance the mental energies to feel less scattered and feel more 'grounded' or rooted.

Standing Mountain Pose *(Tadasana)*

Stand behind the chair with the feet hip-width apart with the hands on the chair top. Have the toes pointing forward. Align the head so that it is centered over the spine. Balance the weight equally on the feet between the right and left foot and front and backs of the feet. Hold and breathe for 1 minute. Release the hands, and bring them alongside the legs or in prayer pose, if you feel stable and balanced. Hold and breathe 5x.

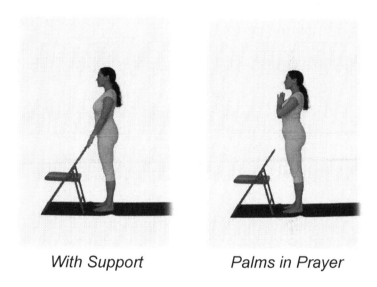

With Support   *Palms in Prayer*

Benefits: Increases concentration, balance and stability (in the body and mind), and allows us to feel a connection to the earth and sky. Helps balance the mental energies.

Seated Gentle Lunge Pose

Bring your hands under one knee. Inhale and lift your knee towards your chest. Lift the belly towards the thigh, keeping the spine tall. Exhale when you lower. Switch legs. Repeat 3x or take 3 to 5 deep breaths while holding the leg on each side.

Variations from Seated Gentle Lunge:

Knee Circles: Make circles in the air with your knee. Switch directions then sides.

Leg Stretch: Stretch your leg out, keeping the hand under the knee for support.

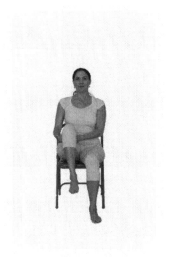

Seated Gentle Lunge

Benefits: Eases hip and low back tension. The Leg Stretch variation stretches the back of the legs.

Seated High Lunge Pose/Horse Rider's Pose
(Ashva Sanchalanasana)

Sit facing the right side of the chair with your right waist facing the back of the chair. Place the right thigh fully on the chair, and release all or part of the left buttocks off the chair. Keep your right hand on the chair back for support and balance assistance. If you are able and comfortable, extend the left leg back into High Lunge Pose.

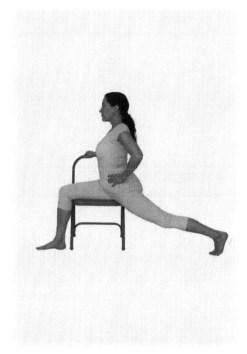

Seated High Lunge Pose

Benefits: Strengthens the legs, assists with balance and opens the hips.

Seated High Lunge Pose Arm Variation
(Ashva Sanchalanasana)

From High Lunge Pose (see previous page) inhale as you lift your left arm up. Hold and breathe for 1 to 5 slow, deep, rhythmic breaths. Switch sides.

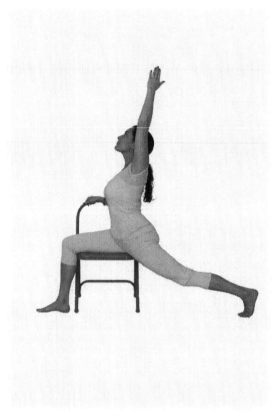

Seated High Lunge Pose Variation

Benefits: Strengthens the legs, increases balance and concentration and opens the hips.

Standing Supported High Lunge/Horse Rider's Pose
(Ashva Sanchalanasana)

From the Standing Warrior 1 Pose (p. 62) or the Standing Warrior II Pose (p. 64) come into High Lunge Pose by curling the back toes under, so that the toes are facing forward towards the chair. You can also come into this posture from Downward Facing Dog (p. 68). From Downward Facing Dog step one foot forward and lift the heart and head. Switch sides.

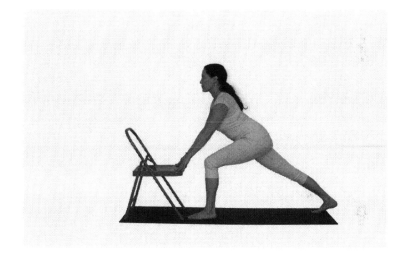

Standing Lunge Pose

Benefits: Strengthens the legs, stretches the back calf muscle and opens the hips.

Standing High Lunge Pose/Horse Rider's Pose
(Ashva Sanchalanasana)

Stand behind the chair. Step your right foot back 3 to 4 feet. Have the back toes curled under, facing the chair. Hold on to the chair back for support, or, if able, inhale as you lift one or both arms overhead. Repeat 2 to 5x or hold steady 2 to 5 slow, deep breaths.

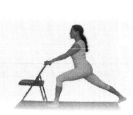 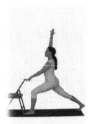 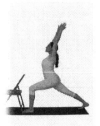

With Support   *One Arm Up*   *Both Arms Up*

Benefits: This pose increases mobility of the hip joint and can ease hip and low back pain. With the arms overhead according to BKS Iyengar in Light on Yoga-it may also help strengthen the heart and tone the side waist. *See references.

Precautions: For knee injuries or balance concerns, try the standing or Seated Lunge Pose (p. 44) or Seated Warrior I *Pose* (p.60) instead of this one. You can also place the back knee on the floor if able, with the hands on the chair base. Place the back knee on a blanket for more comfort.

Seated Powerful Pose *(Utkatasana)*

Press the hands into the chair arms or chair base and lift your body up and down. Have the toes pointing forward and keep the knees facing the toes (trying not to let the knees move towards each other). Repeat 5x. Inhale as you lift and exhale as you lower. Hold the posture with the hands on the hips or reach them overhead for 2 to 5 slow, deep breaths.

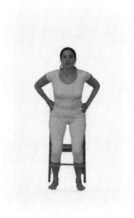 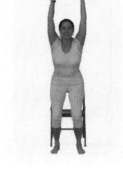

Hands on the Hips   *Hands Overhead*

Benefits: This is called the Powerful Pose in Sanskrit (commonly called the Chair Pose), because it brings great strength to the body (and mind). It strengthens the legs, arms and core. This pose can help prevent falls and keeps the body strong to get up and down from chairs, bed, baths and walkers. It also aids general movements.

Precautions: For shoulder discomfort, keep the hands on the hips, in front of you with the hands in line with the shoulders or along side the legs. For knee discomfort, remain seated and lift the arms only.

Standing Powerful Pose *(Utkatasana)*

Stand behind the chair. Hold on to the chair back with the feet hip-width apart and the toes pointing forward with the knees facing the toes. Exhale as you bend the knees. Try not to let the knees collapse in towards each other. Hold the body in this posture for 2 to 3 deep breaths, or go in and out 3 to 5x. Keep the shoulders relaxed.

If able, lift one hand at a time (or both hands) off the chair and hold for 1 to 3 slow, deep breaths. Switch sides.

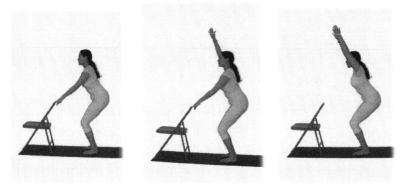

Hands on Chair   One Hand Up   Both Hands Up

Benefits: This is called the Powerful Pose in Sanskrit (commonly called the Chair Pose), because it brings great strength to the body (and mind). It strengthens the legs, arms and core. This pose helps prevent falls and keeps the body strong to get up and down from chairs, bed, baths, walkers, and for other daily activities. *See reference section for evidence-based studies.

Precautions: For shoulder pain, bring the hands on the hips. For knee pain raise the arms only.

Seated Crescent Moon Pose *(Chandrasana)*

Sit tall with the head centered over the spine. Inhale as you lift the left arm up and curve the spine to the right, in a crescent shape. You can also bring the palms together, or interlock the fingers overhead. Keep the buttocks on the chair evenly as you lean to the side. Hold for 1-5 slow, deep breaths. Switch sides.

With Props: Pull the belt apart overhead with your hands as you curve the spine to one side. For arm resistance, pull the belt apart strongly while you keep the shoulders relaxed. Hold for 1-5 slow, deep breaths. Switch sides.

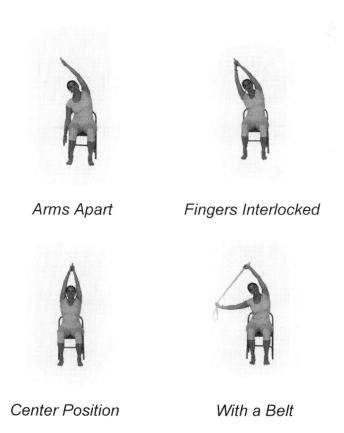

Arms Apart   *Fingers Interlocked*

Center Position   *With a Belt*

Benefits: Stretches the spine and stretches and tones the waist.

Standing Crescent Moon Pose *(Chandrasana)*

Stand tall with the feet hip-width apart and the toes pointing towards the chair or turn your body (legs and feet included) to the side with your right waist facing the chair back. Place the right hand on the chair top for support. Balance the weight on both feet as evenly as you can. Inhale your left arm up, and lean to the right, keeping the weight even on the feet. Switch sides. If able, release both hands off the chair top, and try the posture as you balance. For a deeper stretch through the lower back, keep more weight on the left foot as the left arm reaches up. Reverse for the right side (put more weight on the right foot as the right arm is up).

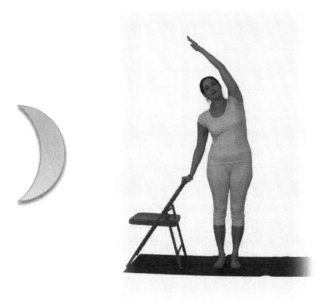

Standing Cresent Moon

Benefits: Stretches the side body and helps tone the waist. The standing version helps strengthen the legs and promotes an increased awareness and sense of balance (physically and mentally).

REFLECTIONS

Take a few moments to practice some of the warms ups. Pause and see how your body, mind and energy level feels afterwards. The warm ups alone can be repeated a few times as your main practice. Or continue on with your practice as you do some rounds of the sun salutations as suggested on the following pages. Take a break and rest if you need.

SUN SALUTATION *(SURYA NAMASKAR)*

Gayatri Mantra (often chanted at sunrise)

ॐ भूर्भुवः स्वः Om Bhur bhuva swaha

तत् सवितुर्वरेण्यं Tat savitur Varenyam

भर्गो देवस्य धीमहि Bhargo Devasya Dhimahi

ह धियो यो नः प्रचोदयात् Dhio yo nah Prachodayat

"AUM -we realize ourselves as manifestation of the Three Worlds and the Beyond; we contemplate the Spiritual Sun that begins to manifest in us in its Perfect Form. We meditate on its Highest Light granting us Wisdom and Bliss. Let it enlighten us with the Light of its Truth." *

*Translation by the Sri Aurobindo Center of Integral Yoga

Sun Salutation Mantras

Om Mitraaya Namaha
Who is friendly to all

Om Ravaye Namaha
The shining one, the radiant one

Om Suryaya Namaha
Who dispels darkness and brings activity

Om Bhaanave Namaha
One who is illuminated, bright one

Om Khagaya Namaha
Who is all pervading, one who moves through the sky

Om Pooshne Namaha
Giver of nourishment & fulfillment

Om Hiranyagarbhaaya Namah
Who has a brilliant golden color

Om Mareechaye Namaha
The giver of infinite rays of light

Om Aadityaaya Namaha
Producer of Everything

Om Aarkaaya Namaha
One who is the Healer and inspires Awe in All

Om Bhaaskaraya Namaha
Giver of wisdom and cosmic illumination

Sun Salutations *(Surya Namaskar)*

Chair Yoga Sun Salutations are postures that flow together, moving with the rhythm of the breath. This is based on a traditional, standing yoga Sun Salutation. Traditionally, they were done to honor the rising and setting of the sun and to create heat in the body, flexibility and overall wellness.

The sun sustains our planet. Without the sun, we would not exist on earth. Here, we can take time to honor the actual sun and to honor the elements of heat, warmth and energy within.

Yoga Sun Salutations can be done using chairs as a seated or standing support tool. Match the seated and standing Sun Salutations to the rhythm of the breath. If you need extra support standing, you can put a second chair in front of you, and one behind you for added assistance to your balance. Rest as needed.

You can do this as a flowing sequence with one breath per movement (as a moving meditation) or hold each posture for 3 to 5 deep breaths or as you feel comfortable. You can alternate between the seated and standing versions, as you need. When you are finished, sit quietly and relax in your chair for 5 to 8 slow, deep breaths. Observe the heart rate (which may speed up from Sun Salutations). Observe the temperature of the body (which may heat up from this sequence). Allow the heart and body to relax. See the Seated and Standing Sun Salutations on the following pages.

Benefits: Increases mobility, energy, flexibility, circulation and endurance, brings vitality at the beginning or middle of the day, or is calming to unwind at the end of the day. It is most powerful when done at sunrise or sunset.

Seated SunLight Chair Yoga Sun Salutations

1. Bring the hands to Prayer Pose in front of the heart center.

2. Inhale as you stretch the arms up overhead.

3. Exhale as you bend forward.

4. Inhale to roll the spine up, and then hold the right leg under the right knee for Lunge Pose. Exhale as you lower the leg.

5. Inhale to lift the left knee towards the chest. Exhale as you lower the leg.

6. Inhale Cobra Pose.

7. Exhale relax.

8. Inhale as you bring the hands up overhead. Imagine you are gathering energy *(prana)* from the sun.

9. Exhale and bring the palms back to Prayer Pose.

    Repeat 3 to 8x. *See photos on the next page.*

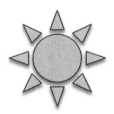

Seated Sun Salutations

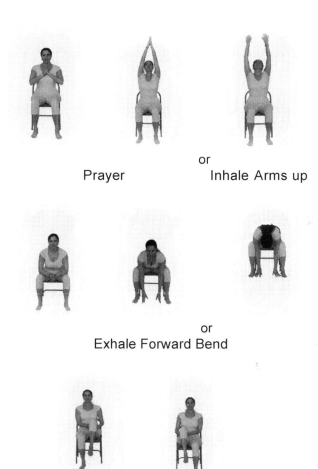

Prayer   or   Inhale Arms up

or
Exhale Forward Bend

Inhale Lunge. Exhale Lower. Switch sides.

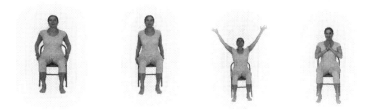

Inhale Cobra. Exhale. Inhale Arms Up. Exhale Prayer.

Standing SunLight Chair Yoga Sun Salutations

1. Stand in Mountain Pose behind a chair. Keep the hands on the chair for balance or bring the palms in Prayer Pose.

2. Inhale as you stretch the arms up overhead.

3. Exhale as you bend forward, resting the head on the forearms on the chair top, the hands on the chair top or chair base.

4. Inhale as you step one leg back to Warrior I Pose (the back foot is flat on the ground with the toes pointing 45 degrees towards the front foot). Or, go into Proud Warrior or High Lunge Pose (the back toes are curled under with the toes facing the chair). Exhale relax.

5. Inhale one or both arms up. Exhale as you lower the arms. Switch sides or hold both arms overhead for an extra breath.

6. Inhale as you step forward into Mountain Pose (or Downward Facing Dog). Exhale. Switch legs and inhale as you step into Warrior I, Proud Warrior or High Lunge Pose on the other side.

7. Exhale to Mountain Pose.

8. Inhale as you lift the heart into an upper back bend (Cobra Pose). Exhale relax.

9. Inhale as you lift the arms up. Imagine you are gathering *(prana)* energy from the sun.

10. Exhale and bring the palms back to Prayer.

    Repeat 3 to 8x. See *photos on the next page.*

Standing Sun Salutations

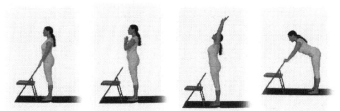

Inhale Mountain. Exhale Prayer. Inhale Arms up. Exhale Forward Bend (with the head up or resting as in the photos below).

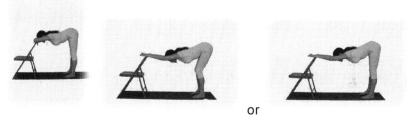

or

Forward Bend Options: The hand or head can rest on the chair top, with the knees bent or straight.

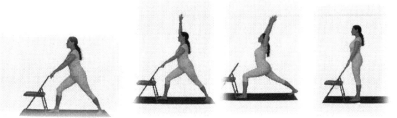

Inhale Warrior or High Lunge. Exhale relax. Inhale and lift one arm up. Exhale, lower. Inhale and lift the other arm up. Exhale, lower. Inhale and lift both arms up. Exhale, lower and step forward. Switch legs and repeat. Inhale Mountain. Exhale.

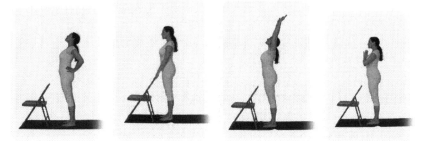

Inhale Cobra. Exhale Mountain. Inhale Arms Up. Exhale Prayer Pose. Repeat this cycle 2-8x.

Seated Postures

Seated Warrior I Pose *(Virabhadrasana)*

Copy the same arm movements as the standing versions
(p.62-66). To add the leg movements in the chair, instead
of stepping one leg back, stretch one foot out in front of
you (as in the photo below), coordinating the leg and the
arm movements with the breath.

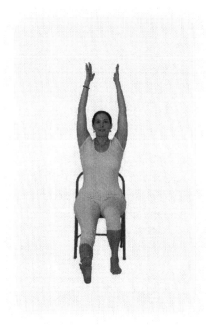

Arms Overhead

Benefits: Strengthens the arms and legs, improves focus,
balance and concentration. *For more benefits see the
reference section.

Seated Warrior II *(Virabhadrasana)*

Stretch the left leg straight and out to the left, keeping the left toes facing forward. The right leg remains bent with the knee and toes turned to the right. Balance the weight on the feet. Stretch the arms out to the side, as in the photo below. Look towards the right shoulder, gazing over the right middle finger. Relax the shoulders and enjoy 3 to 5 slow, deep breaths. Switch sides and repeat.

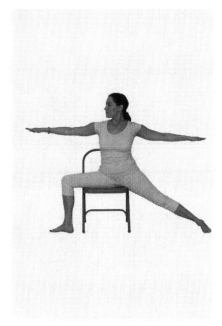

Seated Warrior II

Benefits: Strengthens the arms and legs and opens the hips. This can help prevent falls by making you aware of the balance in your feet. Improves focus, balance and concentration.

Standing Postures

Warrior I Pose with Support *(Virabhadrasana)*

Stand behind the chair. Place your hands on the top of the chair back for support. Step one leg back, and turn your back toes in (about 45 degrees) towards the chair. Exhale as you bend the front knee (do not bend the knee further than it being over the front heel). Hold for 2-5 slow, deep breaths or bend the front knee as you exhale, and inhale as you straighten the leg, going back and forth 2 to 5x.

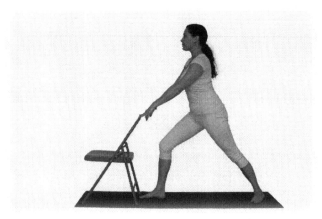

Warrior I With Support

Benefits: Strengthens the arms and legs. This standing version can help prevent falls by being aware of the balance in the feet. Improves focus, balance and concentration.

Warrior I Pose with Arm(s) Up *(Virabhadrasana)*

From Warrior I with Support, inhale as you lift one arm overhead or as far as comfortable. Exhale as you lower the arm. Switch sides. Repeat 2 to 4x or hold and breath 2 to 4 deep breaths on each side. Try it with both arms up. Repeat 2x.

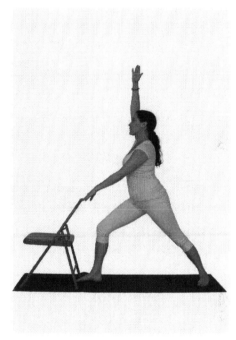

With One Arm Up

Benefits: Strengthens the arms and legs. This standing version can help prevent falls by being aware of the balance in the feet. Improves focus, balance and concentration.

Precautions: For knee or ankle discomfort, you can remain seated and lift the arms only or try Seated Warrior I (p. 60).

Standing Warior II *(Virabhadrasana)*

Stand behind the chair and step your left foot back. Place the left toes to face the chair 45 degrees by rotating the back thighbone slightly inward. Balance the weight equally on both feet. Open the hips as you stretch the left arm towards the wall behind you. Look over your right shoulder, if the neck is comfortable. If able lift the right hand off the chair and stretch it forward. Focus the eyes over the right middle finger. Hold for 2 to 6 slow, deep breaths. Feel the feet firm on the earth.

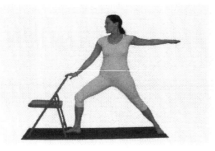

With Hand On Chair

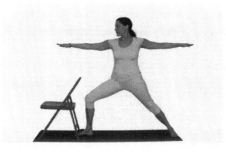

Warrior II

Benefits: Strengthens the legs and arms and improves balance. Improves mental focus and prepares the mind to meet goals with the strength, balance and peace of a spiritual warrior (physically and mentally).

Precautions: For instability, place your back heel against a wall for support. Or try Seated Warrior I (p. 60)

Reverse Warrior *(Virabhadrasana)*

From Warrior II (p. 64) place the left hand on the left leg, and lift the right arm up by the right ear. Curve the spine back towards your back leg. Hold for 3 to 5 slow, deep breaths. Switch sides and repeat.

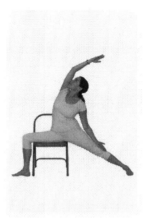

Seated Reverse Warrior

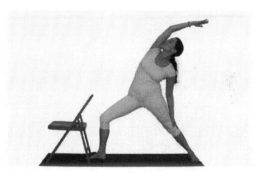

Standing Reverse Warrior

Benefits: Strengthens the arms and legs, opens the hips and side ribs and stretches the side body. Helps feel as if you have more room to breathe (mentally and physically).

Precautions: For joint instability, place your back heel against a wall for support or do Seated Warrior I (p. 60).

Proud Warrior

Inhale and lift one or both arms overhead. Exhale to lower the arms. If able, hold the arms overhead for 3 to 5 slow, deep breaths. Feel the heart area lifting up towards the sky.

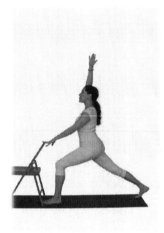

One Arm Up

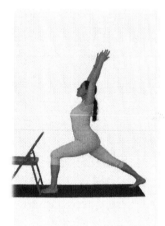

Both Arms Up

Benefits: Strengthens the arms and legs and opens the hips. This standing version can help prevent falls by causing you to be aware of the balance in the feet. Improves focus, balance and concentration. This pose can create a feeling of joy and uplifts you as the heart area opens. Imagine you are saying "yes" to life and longevity.

Precautions: If there is ankle, knee or hip joint discomfort, try Warrior I (p.62) or Seated Warrior I (p. 60).

Intense Side Stretch Pose *(Parsvottanasana)*

Stand behind the chair in Mountain Pose (p.43). Step your right foot back. Rotate the back thighbone inwards so that the back toes face the chair at 45-degree angle. Balance the weight equally on both feet. Inhale as you stretch the spine towards the sky. Exhale as you bend forward. Stretch the spine towards the chair, resting the hands on the top of the chair back or chair base. Relax the shoulders and square the hips (gently move the left outer thigh/hip back and the right outer thigh/hip forward). Hold for 1 to 5 slow, deep breaths.

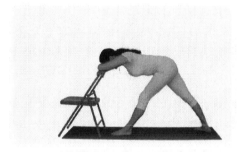

Head on the Chair

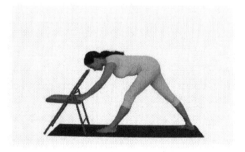

Hands on the Chair

Benefits: Stretches and strengthens the legs and improves balance.

Precautions: For knee, hamstring or hip injuries, softly bend one or both knees. There should be no strain. For vertigo, dizziness or blood pressure concerns, keep the head up and the back foot against a wall for support.

"Chair or Desk" Downward Facing Dog
(Adho Mukha Savasana)

Stand tall in front of your chair or desk with the feet hip-width apart and the toes pointing forward. Exhale and fold forward from the hips. Place the hands on the chair top or base (or desk). Bend your knees at first, and, if able, straighten the legs (one at a time or both) - or rest your forearms and head on the chair top for more support. If comfortable, rest your hands on the chair base or bottom of the chair (or desk legs). You can also let go of the chair and release the head and spine into a full forward bend. Hold for 1 to 5 slow, deep breaths. To come out, bend the knees and place the hands on the chair or desk top, lift the heart and the head slowly and roll or rise up mindfully.

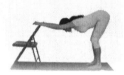

With Knees Bent

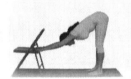

Hands on Chair Base

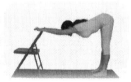

With Straight Legs

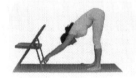

Hands on Chair Bottom

Benefits: Stretches the back and legs and calms the mind.

Precautions: For low back discomfort, vertigo or dizziness and third trimester pregnancy, keep your hands on the chair top and the head upright (as needed).

Standing Wide-Legged Forward Bend
(Prasarita Padottanasana)

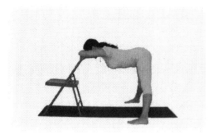

Head on Forearms

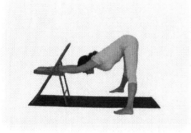

Stand with your feet farther than hip-width apart and the toes pointing forward. Inhale, stand tall and lift the heart. Exhale and fold forward, resting the hands on a second chair top, base or lower chair bars.

Hands on Chair Base

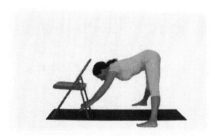

Hands on Chair Lower Legs

Benefits: Stretches and strengthens the back and legs, brings awareness in the feet, opens the hips and is calming.

Precautions: Keep your head up for vertigo, or blood pressure issues. Bend the knees and/or keep the spine upright for any lower back discomfort.

Revolved Standing Wide-Legged Forward Bend
(Paravritta Prasarita Padottanasana)

Stand with your feet wider than hip-width apart and the toes pointing forward. Inhale, stand tall and lift the heart. Exhale and fold forward, resting the hands on a second chair top, base or lower chair bars. Only go as far as comfortable. Place your left hand on the left hip and gently twist the spine to the left. Keep the head centered or, if comfortable, gently look up towards the sky over the left shoulder. Hold as long as comfortable. Switch sides.

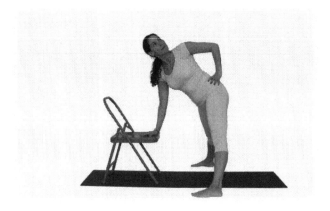

Revolved Standing Wide Legged Forward Bend

Benefits: Stretches and strengthens the back and legs, increases awareness in the feet, opens the hips and is calming. Twists can also ease and balance the digestive system.

Precautions: Keep your head centered if you have vertigo or experience dizziness. Bend the knees and keep the spine upright for back pain or injuries that are aggravated by this pose. If you are pregnant, twist from above the upper ribs only.

Backbends

Seated Cobra Pose *(Bhujangasana)*

Bring the hands towards the hips, or place them on the upper thighs. Lift your chest bone (sternum) without overarching the low back. Keep a neutral pelvis, feeling the low back comfortable, not arched nor collapsed. Maintain the head centered over the spine. Look up with the eyes and chin slightly, relaxing the neck and shoulders. You can also bring your hands to the hips, and move the elbows towards each other behind you. Take 2 to 4 deep breaths.

Bring the hands under or on the back of the chair base, as in the second photo below. Lift the heart area as you take 3 to 5 slow, deep breaths. Or repeat the posture 3 times: inhale as you lift the heart area and exhale as you release the posture.

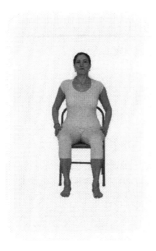

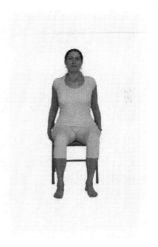

Hand on the Thighs   *Hands on Chair Base*

Benefits: Opens the upper back, chest and shoulders, eases dullness and can help ease depression. It can also bring relief (emotional and/or physical). from slouching in a chair or wheelchair.

Seated Cobra Variation *(Bhujangasana)*

Interlock the fingers behind your back. If it is more comfortable, place the hands on the lower back or hips instead. Lift the heart area as you gently stretch the hands towards the earth. Take 3 to 5 deep breaths. Release and relax.

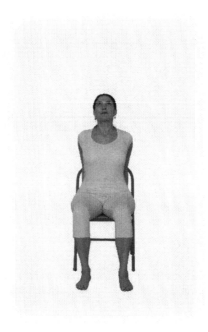

Fingers Interlocked

Benefits: Releases computer-related, travel-related and general tension in the upper back and improves posture. This pose counteracts the slouching position from sitting for long periods in a chair, at your desk or on airplanes and increases general feelings of vitality. This can be a useful a prenatal backbend variation and post surgery option. (Cobra Pose is traditionally done lying on the stomach).

Seated Half Bow Pose *(Ardha Dhanurasana)*

From Seated High Lunge Pose (p. 45), bend the left knee and grab hold of the left foot or ankle with your left hand. You can also use a belt for assistance. To create a deeper back bend, gently press the left foot or ankle into the left hand (or belt) and the left hand into the foot simultaneously. Hold for 1 to 3 deep breaths. Switch sides.

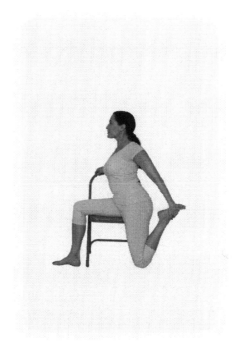

Half Bow Pose

Benefits: Opens the upper back, heart area and hip. Stretches the front of the back thigh (quadriceps).

Precautions: For knee injuries or discomfort do not do Bow Pose or High Lunge Pose. Instead try the Seated Lunge Pose (p.44) or Seated Warrior I (p. 60). Do not strain or hold longer than you are comfortable.

Standing Cobra Pose *(Bhujangasana)*

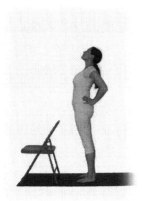

Hands on Low Back

Stand with the feet hip width apart. Place the hands on the hips or lower back. Move the elbows towards each other behind you. Lift the heart towards the sky. Enjoy 1 to 5 deep breaths.

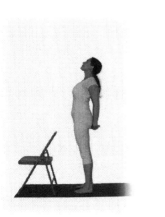

Fingers Interlocked

Interlock your fingers behind the lower back. Inhale as you move the hands towards the earth and lift the heart towards the sky. Keep the pelvis in a neutral position (do not over arch the low back, nor push the hips forward). There should be no pain or strain.

Benefits: Releases tension in the upper back and improves posture. This pose can help ease depression and dullness (in the body and/or mind) It counteracts the rounding of the upper back and shoulders from computer use and sitting for long periods of time. This is a prenatal modification for Cobra Pose (all trimesters).

Standing Locust Pose Variations *(Salabhasana)*

Stand behind the chair with the feet hip-width apart. Balance the weight equally on both feet. Move your tailbone towards the floor as you move the navel area in towards the spine. Lift the spine as you extend one leg/foot back. Keep your toes on the floor, if needed, and your hands on the chair, or release one hand from the chair, and lift the arm overhead. Hold for 3 to 5 slow, deep breaths while stretching the back leg. Switch sides.

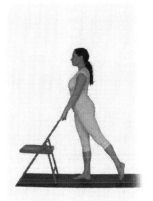   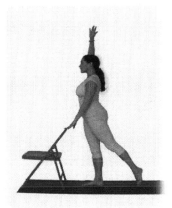

With Support   *One Arm Up*

Balancing Locust

While in Locust Pose, inhale as you lift both arms up. Exhale as you lower. Repeat 2x. Or hold and balance with both arms overhead. Enjoy 3 to 5 slow, deep breaths as you hold the posture. Keep the shoulders relaxed and the area below the navel moving slightly in towards the spine so that the pelvis is in a neutral position.

Benefits: Strengthens the legs and buttocks. Increases the range of motion in the hips. This is a prenatal modification for the Locust Pose (all trimesters).

Spinal Twists

Seated Spinal Twist *(Ardha Matsyendrasana)*

Inhale as you sit tall. Exhale as you twist to one side. Keep the head centered over the spine and twist gently and evenly throughout the entire spine. You can cross your legs fully or just the ankles. See the next page for photos showing details about how to get into the posture.

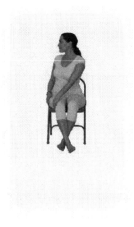

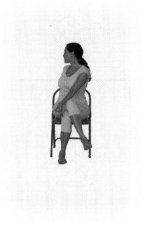

Ankles Crossed   *Legs Crossed*

Benefits: Releases back tension, helps the digestive organs and calms the nervous system. Increases spinal flexibility.

Precautions: If pregnant, for all twists, do not twist through the torso (belly). Twist only from the area above the ribcage (all trimesters). For whiplash or neck pain, keep the head facing forward or as comfortable.

Getting into the Spinal Twist

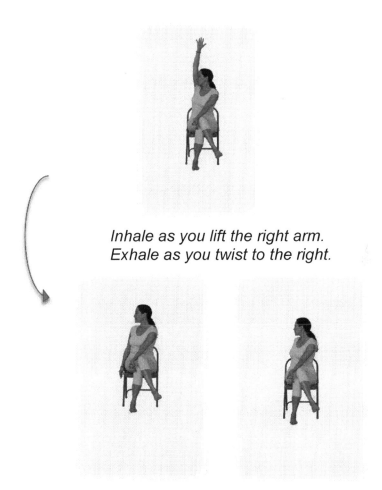

Inhale as you lift the right arm.
Exhale as you twist to the right.

Arm by the Chair Side   Arm by the Chair Back

Breath Pattern: Inhale as you lengthen the spine (sit tall).
Exhale as you gently twist. Hold for 1 to 5 deep breaths.

Seated Spinal Twist (Side Facing) *(Bharadvajasana)*

Turn your body and legs to the side of the chair with the side of your body facing the chair back. Keep your feet on the floor, hip width apart. Inhale as you sit tall. Exhale as you twist towards the chair back. Hold for 3 to 5 breaths or go in and out of the posture 3 to 5x. Example: Inhale as you sit tall. Exhale as you twist. Repeat 3 to 5x on both sides.

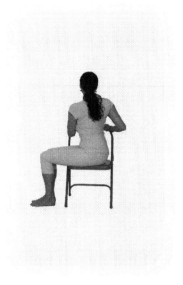

Side Facing Spinal Twist

Benefits: Releases back tension, helps the digestive organs, calms the nervous system, increases spinal flexibility.

Spinal Twist With A Belt

Hold a belt between the hands overhead. Pull the belt apart to create some resistance. Inhale and sit tall. Exhale as you twist to the right, keeping the head centered over the spine. Inhale as you return to center. Exhale and twist to the left. Repeat 3 to 5x or hold for 1 to 3 deep breaths on each side.

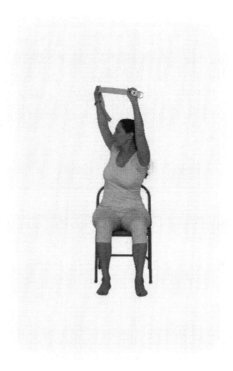

With a Belt

Benefits: Eases back tension and helps the digestive system. Spinal twists are also calming for the nervous system and the mind. Pulling the belt apart creates resistance, which activates and strengthens the upper arms.

Seated Wide-Legged Twist With 3 Chairs
(Upavishta Konasana)

Separate the feet wider than hip width apart, or as wide as comfortable and place each foot on a separate chair. Keep your buttocks on the chair base. Inhale as you sit tall. Exhale, as you gently twist to the left, resting your right arm on your inner right or left thigh. Look towards the left shoulder, or keep the head centered if that is more comfortable. Repeat the breathing pattern like before, and hold for 1 to 5 slow, deep breaths (inhale as you lengthen, exhale as you relax and twist). Switch sides.

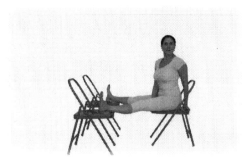

Wide Legged Twist

Benefits: Stretches the spine, and legs, strengthens the quadriceps, helps the digestive system and eases back tension.

Precautions: Keep your head centered for neck pain, whiplash or dizziness. If you are pregnant, twist only from above the upper ribs.

Seated Wide-Legged Forward Bend Twist Variation

Inhale as you sit tall. Exhale as you twist the spine and head gently to the right. Rest your left elbow on the left thigh or on the inside of the left lower leg (or floor). Bring the right hand to the right hip, chair base behind you or extend it up towards the sky. Hold for 1 to 3 slow breaths. Gaze skywards if comfortable. Switch sides.

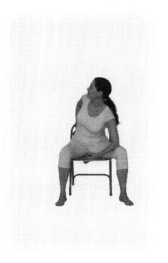   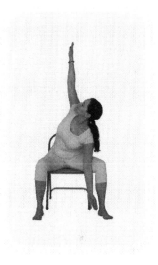

Arm on the Thigh   *Arm in the Air*

Benefits: Eases back tension and benefits the digestive system.

Precautions: Keep your head centered if you are dizzy or have neck pain. If you are pregnant, twist only from above the upper ribs.

Forward Bends

Seated Forward Bend *(Uttanasana)*

Place the feet hip width apart. Inhale as you sit tall. Exhale as you fold at the hips into a forward bend. Keep your buttocks on the chair base.

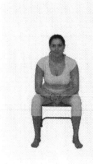

Arms on Thighs

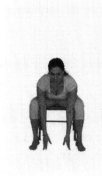
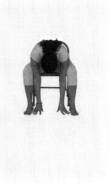

Head Up   *Hands to Floor*

Benefits: Stretches the back and legs and is calming.

Precautions: Keep your head up for vertigo, dizziness or blood pressure issues.

Extended Leg Forward Bend *(Paschimotanasa)*

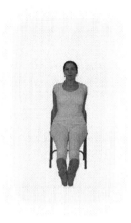

Both Legs

Hold on to the chair back or base. Stretch the legs out, and pull the toes towards the face. Exhale as you bend forward from the hips, keeping the buttocks evenly pressing into the chair base. Keep the sternum (chest bone) lifting and the spine lengthening.

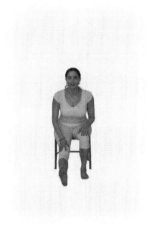

One Leg

Head to Knee Pose
(Janu Sirsasana)

Try the same posture as above, with only one leg stretched out. The other knee should be bent with the foot flat on the floor.

Benefits: Stretches the back and legs and calms the mind.

Precautions: Bend the knees softly if you need to ease any strain in the hamstrings or behind the knees.

Seated Forward Bend (*Paschimottanasana*)

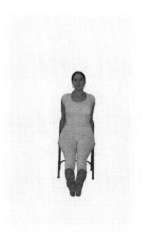

With One Chair

With one chair, hold on to back of the chair base, and extend your legs. Inhale as you sit tall. Exhale and fold forward.

With two chairs, inhale to sit tall. As you exhale, reach towards the toes (or use a belt wrapped around the feet). Lift the sternum (chest bone) to create length to the spine (avoid collapsing the upper back). Hold for 1 to 5 slow, deep breaths.

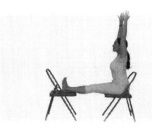

With Two Chairs:

Inhale, Arms Up.

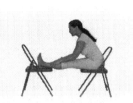

Exhale, Bend Forward.

Benefits: Stretches the back and legs and calms the mind.

Precautions: Do not bend forward if there is any pain or discomfort. Be comfortable and never overstretch.

Head to Knee Pose With 2 Chairs (*Janu Sirsasana*)

Use two chairs for this posture.

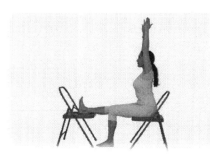

Inhale, Arms Up.

Exhale, Bend Forward.

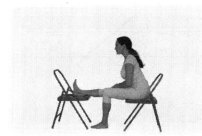

Sit tall, away from the chair back. Lift your right foot onto a second chair placed 2 to 3 feet in front of you. Inhale as you sit tall. Exhale, bend at the hips and reach towards the right thigh, shin or toes. Use a belt or strap around the right toes for support. Lift the sternum (chest bone) and spine. Hold for 1 to 5 deep breaths. Switch sides.

Benefits: Stretches the back and legs and calms the mind.

Precautions: Keep your head up for vertigo, dizziness or blood pressure issues. Keep the spine upright (not bending forward) as in the first photo for low back pain or injuries. For hamstring or knee injuries, softly bend the straight leg.

If you do not have two chairs available or are unable to lift your legs, try the Seated Head to Knee Pose Using 1 Chair (p. 83).

Head to Knee Pose Twist Variation

Sit tall away from the chair back. Lift your right foot onto a second chair placed 2 to 3 feet out in front of you. Inhale as you sit tall. Exhale as you bend forward and gently twist to the left, touching the left inner or outer thigh with your right hand or right outer upper arm (or with the hands in Prayer Pose). Hold for 1 to 5 deep breaths. Switch sides.

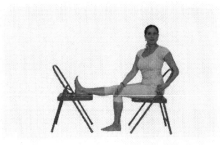

Hand on the Outer Thigh

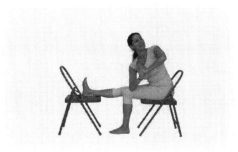

Elbow on the Outer Thigh

Benefits: Improves digestion, releases back, shoulder and mental tension and calms the mind.

Precautions: Keep the spine upright (not bending forward or twisting) if there is lower back pain or if you are pregnant (second and third trimesters).

Seated Wide-Legged Forward Bend
(Upavistha Konasana)

Separate the feet wider than hip-width apart, or as wide as is comfortable. Keep your buttocks on the chair base. Inhale as you sit tall. Exhale as you fold at the hips into a forward bend. Rest the arms on the thighs. You can also place your hands on a block or second chair in front of you. Hold for 1-5 slow, deep breaths.

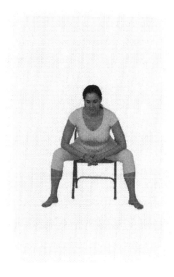

With the Head Up

Benefits: Extends the spine and back body, releases the groins, opens the hips and calms the mind.

Precautions: For lower back pain or injuries, keep the spine upright and only bend forward (if at all) as much as comfortable. Focus on extending the spine on the inhalation and relaxing the shoulders on the exhalation. Keep your head up for vertigo, dizziness or blood pressure issues.

Seated Wide-Legged Forward Bend
(Upavistha Konasana)

Separate the feet wider than hip-width apart, or as wide as is comfortable. Keep your buttocks on the chair base. Inhale as you sit tall. Exhale as you fold at the hips into a forward bend. Reach the hands towards the earth (floor). You can also place your hands on a block or second chair in front of you. Hold for 1-5 slow, deep breaths.

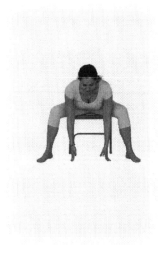

Hands to the Floor

Benefits: Stretches the back of the legs, extends the spine, releases the groins, opens the hips and calms the mind.

Precautions: For lower back pain or injuries, keep the spine upright and only bend forward (if at all) as much as comfortable. Focus on extending the spine on the inhalation and relaxing the shoulders on the exhalation. Keep the head up for dizziness or blood pressure issues.

Seated Wide-Legged Forward Bend With 3 Chairs
(Upavistha Konasana)

Separate the feet wider than hip-width apart, or as wide as is comfortable. Lift one leg up at a time onto the second and third chair, placed in front of you. Bring the chairs closer together if there is any strain. Keep your buttocks and upper thighs firmly pressing into the chair base. Inhale as you sit tall. Rest the hands on the legs or reach the arms up as you inhale. Hold for 1 to 5 slow, deep breaths.

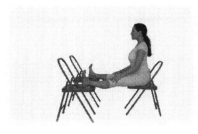

Inhale, Sitting Tall

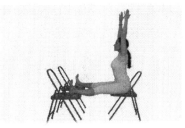

With Arms Up

Exhale as you fold at the hips into a forward bend. Rest the arms on the thighs, or if able, reach the hands towards the toes. You can also place your hands on the base of the chairs in front of you. Hold for 1 to 5 deep breaths. Switch sides.

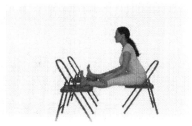

Exhale, Bend Forward.

Benefits: Stretches the back and legs, and calms the mind.

Precautions: Keep the head up for dizziness or blood pressure issues. Keep the spine upright (not bending forward) if there is any lower back pain or discomfort.

Bound Angle Pose Forward Bend
(*Baddha Konasana*)

Sit tall in a chair. Lift one foot up at a time onto a second chair placed in front of you and bring the feet together. Relax the knees out to the sides. Keep your buttocks on the chair base. Inhale as you sit tall. Exhale as you fold at the hips into a forward bend. Rest the arms on the thighs, or if able, hold on to the ankles or toes. Inhale, extend and lengthen the spine. Exhale as you fold forward. Hold for 1 to 5 deep breaths.

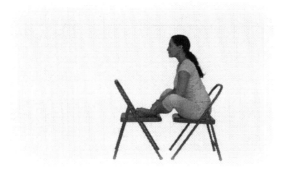

Bound Angle Pose With 2 Chairs

Benefits: Stretches the spine and open the hips. This pose can ease prenatal and menstrual discomfort.

Precautions: Keep your head up for vertigo, dizziness or blood pressure issues. Keep the spine upright (not bending forward) for lower back pain or related injuries.

One-Legged Pigeon Pose *(Eka Pada Kapotasana)*

Sit with the feet hip width apart. Place your right foot on top of your left thigh. Exhale as you bend forward. Keep the sternum (chest bone) lifting and the buttocks releasing into the chair base. Feel the sides of the waist and spine lengthen.

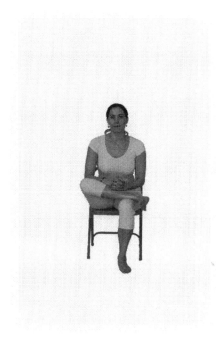

Pigeon Pose

Benefits: Increases the range of motion externally in the hip socket and opens the hips flexors.

Seated Triangle Pose *(Trikonasana)*

Inhale as you stretch your arms away from the heart in a "T" shape. Exhale as you lean to one side. Inhale as you bring the torso back to the center. Exhale as you lean to the other side. If comfortable, when leaning to the right, gently turn the head and spine, twisting from the right ribs towards the left ribs (skywards). Gaze at the left fingers. Repeat 3x or hold for 3 to 5 breaths on each side.

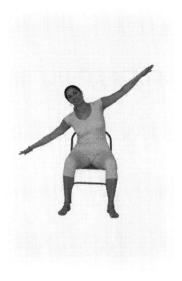

Triangle Pose Seated

Benefits: Stretches the sides of the body and the arms. Flexibility is improved by bending the spine sideways. This posture also helps the mind to focus inward (on the heart area).

Precautions: For neck pain or prenatal variations, keep the spine and head centered (do not twist).

Seated Triangle Pose Variation *(Trikonasana)*

Follow the steps on the previous page for the Triangle Pose. Extend the right leg out to the right and flex the foot. Exhale as you lean to the right with the arms extended. Hold for 1 to 3 slow breaths. Switch sides.

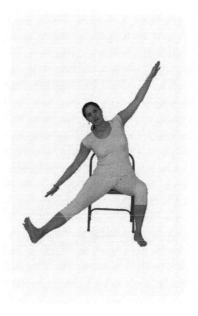

With Leg Extended

Benefits: Stretches the sides of the body, the arms and the extended leg. Flexibility is improved by bending the spine sideways. This posture also helps the mind to focus inward (on the heart area).

Precautions: For neck pain or prenatal variations, keep the spine and head centered (do not twist.).

Standing Extended Triangle Pose *(UtthitaTrikonasana)*

Stand behind the chair. Step your left leg 3 to 4 feet back. Turn your left toes towards the chair (spiral the thighbone inward). Turn the body so that your torso faces to the left. Place the right hand on the top of the chair or chair base (as in the photos below). Inhale. Exhale as you shift your hips to the left and place your left hand on the hip (or stretch your left arm towards the sky). Twist the spine and torso gently to the left (towards the sky). Hold for 3 to 5 deep breaths per side, or inhale to come out and exhale to go into the posture, repeating 3x.

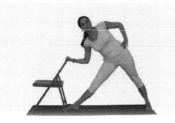

Hands on the Hip and Chair Top

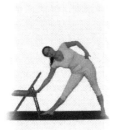 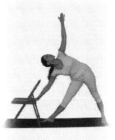

Hand on Chair Base   *Arm Extended*

Benefits: Stretches the sides of the body, strengthens and stretches the legs and opens the hips.

Precautions: If pregnant, twist from above the upper ribs. If you have neck pain, keep the head centered.

Seated Extended Side Angle Pose
(Utthita Parsvakonasana)

Rest your right thigh on the chair base. Stretch the left leg out to the left, with the toes turned in slightly towards the chair. Stretch the arms away from the heart in a lateral "T" shape. Inhale as you sit tall. Exhale, lean to the right resting your right arm on the right thigh, or the right hand on the floor behind the right foot. Stretch the left arm along side the ear (or place it on the left hip). Gaze at the left upper arm. Hold for 1 to 3 deep breaths. Switch sides.

Deepening Alignment: To increase the hip opening, gently guide your right thigh back so that the knee moves towards the little toe side of the right foot. While the thigh moves back, the spine twists gently towards the sky (right ribs moving towards the left ribs or sky).

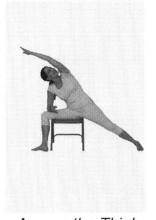

Arm on the Thigh

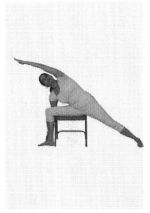

Arm Behind the Leg

Benefits: Stretches the sides of the body and legs and opens the hips.

Precautions: For shoulder discomfort, place the top hand on the top hip or try Seated Warrior II (p. 61). For neck discomfort keep the head looking forward (or down) as in the second photo above.

Standing Extended Side Angle Pose
(Utthita Parsvakonasana)

Place a chair to your right side. Separate your legs 3 to 4 feet apart. Turn your right toes towards the chair (to the right). Place the right hand on the top of the chair or the chair base (where you sit). Inhale. Exhale as you bend the right knee (the knee should not go further than the right heel) and stretch your left arm towards the sky and over the left ear. Hold for 3 to 5 deep breaths per side, or inhale to come out and exhale to go into the posture, repeating 3x.

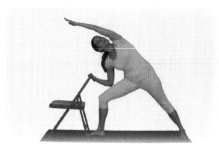

Hand on the Chair Top

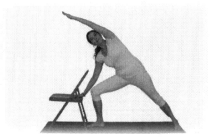

Hand on the Chair Base

Benefits: Stretches the sides of the body, opens the hips and strengthens the legs. Assists in balance awareness to help prevent falls.

Precautions: For shoulder pain, place the top hand on the top hip. There should be no pain in the joints.

Balance Postures

Tree Pose *(Vrksasana)*

Seated: Bring the palms to Prayer Pose. Inhale as you lift your arms up overhead in a "Y" shape or with the palms together. Bring one heel behind the opposite ankle with the toes on floor. Then try to lift your toes on that same foot you placed behind the ankle. Focus the eyes on one point in front of you. Hold and balance for 3 to 5 deep breaths. Switch sides. Or inhale as you go into the pose and exhale as you release. Repeat 3x.

Standing: Stand to the left side of the chair. Hold your right hand on the chair. Place the left heel behind the left ankle, shifting the weight to the right leg and foot. Focus the eyes and mind on one stationary point in front of you. Hold the posture and take 5 deep breaths. Stand tall like a tree.

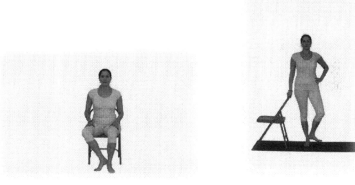

Seated   *Standing*
With the Heel Behind the Ankle

Benefits: Improves balance (physically and emotionally) and mental concentration.

Tree Pose Variations *(Vrksasana)*

From Tree Pose (previous page), place the foot that is behind the ankle to the inside of the opposite shin. Keep the eyes and mind focused on one point. Extend the outer arm to the side or on a diagonal away from the body. Hold for 1 to 5 slow, deep breaths. Switch sides.

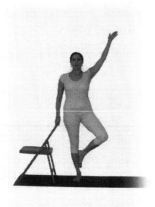

Standing With Foot on Lower Leg and Arm Extended

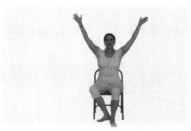

Seated With Foot Behind Ankle and Arms Up

Benefits: Improves balance, concentration and helps prevent falls by bringing awareness to the weight shifts on the feet. The tree symbolizes life and increased vitality.

Tree Pose Variations *(Vrksasana)*

From Tree Pose (previous page), carry the foot that is inside of the opposite shin higher up, towards the inside of the inner thigh, as high as you can comfortably go. Balance and breathe. Focus the eyes on one point. Relax the shoulders, stomach and face. Feel the crown (top) of the head lifting up towards the sky as the standing leg and foot root themselves into the earth. Hold for 1 to 5 deep breaths. Switch sides.

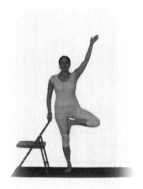

Standing

(With Foot on Inner Thigh)

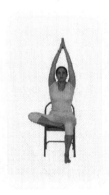

Seated

Benefits: Improves balance, concentration and confidence and helps prevent falls by bringing awareness to the weight shifts on the feet. The tree symbolizes life and can increase your vitality and energy.

Tree Pose *(Vrksasana)*

From either the seated or standing Tree Poses (see previous pages), lift one arm up as you inhale. Exhale as you lower the arm. Switch sides. Repeat 2x. Then lift both arms up overhead and focus the eyes on one point. Breathe and balance for as long as you are comfortable. Keep the shoulders, face and stomach relaxed. Stretch the sides of the body and feel the standing leg and foot rooting into the earth. Switch sides. Come out of the pose to rest.

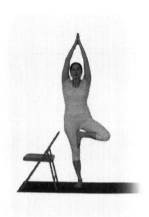   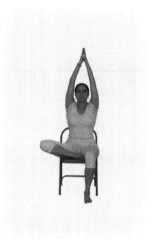

Standing Tree Pose   *Seated Tree Pose*

Benefits: Improves balance, concentration and confidence. It stretches the spine and waist and brings awareness to the weight shifts on the feet, which can help prevent falls. The tree symbolizes life and can increase your vitality and energy.

Warrior III *(Virabhadrasana)*

From Downward Facing Dog (p. 68), lift the left leg up as high as the back, keeping the hipbones facing down. Stretch the left toes and leg back and reach the arms forward simultaneously. Hold and breathe for 1 to 5 deep breaths. Switch Sides.

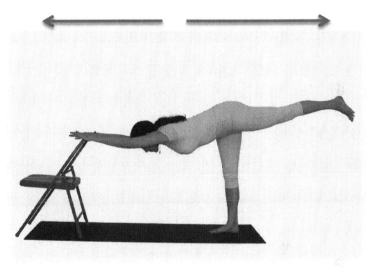

Warrior III With Support

Benefits: Stretches the back and side body. Improves balance, concentration and confidence. The warrior poses also are symbols and reminders of our inner and outer strength and balance, keeping calm and grounded during the inner (and outer) battles of life.

Stork Pose

Stand in Mountain Pose to the left side of the chair with the feet hip-width apart. Place the right hand on the top of the chair back for balance support and the left hand on the left hip. Inhale and lift the left foot off the ground, bringing the knee in line with the left hip joint, or as high as comfortable. Feel the standing leg root itself into the earth. Relax the left upper thigh and shoulder. Hold and breathe for 1 to 5 slow, deep breaths. You can also try to lift the right hand off the chair top onto the right hip and balance.

Arm Lift Variation: At the same time, or once you find your balance, raise the left arm as well. Hold for 1 to 5 slow, deep breaths. Switch sides. Or lift both arms up overhead and hold as long as you are able.

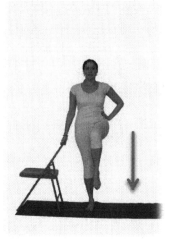
Hand on Hip

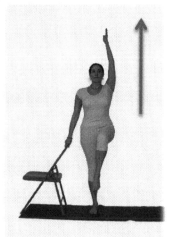
Arm Raised

Benefits: Improves balance and concentration. It stretches the spine and waist and brings awareness to the weight shifts on the feet, which can help prevent falls. This pose also strengthens the standing leg.

Half Moon Pose *(Ardha Chandrasana)*

From Warrior II, Triangle Pose or Extended Side Angle Pose bend the front knee (right knee in these photos). Place the right hand on the chair top or base, keeping the right hand under the right shoulder. The chair or body needs to be placed so that shoulder and hand alignment is kept. Balance on one foot, keeping the right (front) toes pointing towards the chair and the left leg stretched away from the body with the toes pointing forward, as high as the hip (if able). Place the left (top) hand on the left hip or stretch it towards the sky. Hold for 1 to 5 slow breaths as you relax and balance.

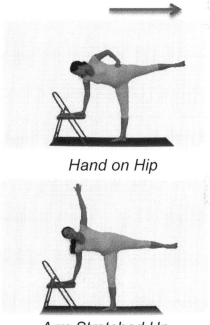

Hand on Hip

Arm Stretched Up

Benefits: Strengthens the legs, improves confidence, concentration and balance. This pose symbolically honors and calls in the moon energy which is cooling, calming and healing in yoga philosophy.

Standing Hand to Foot Pose *(Padangusthasana)*

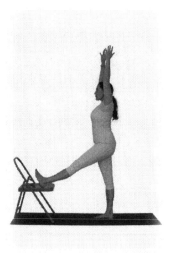

Stand facing the base of the chair. Lift one leg up and place it on the chair. Have the toes and hips pointing forward towards the chair. Inhale and stand tall as you stretch the arms overhead.

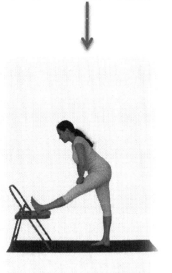

Exhale as you fold forward at the hips, placing your hand on the thigh, shin, foot or toes. Feel the leg stretch gently with no strain. Hold for 3 to 5 deep breaths. Switch sides.

Forward Bend

Benefits: Increases concentration, balance, leg strength and stretches the hamstrings and legs.

Boat Pose *(Navasana)*

Hold on to the chair back or base. Sit tall and away from the chair back. Lift the feet and balance on the sits bones. Inhale to lift out of the lower back and lengthen the spine. If comfortable, lift the feet up in line with the knees. Hold for 1-3 slow, deep breaths. Relax the shoulders and jaw in this pose.

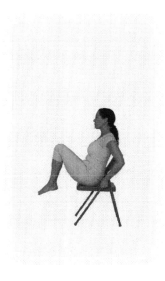

With Knees Bent

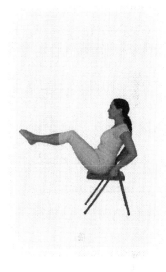

Feet In Line With Knees

Benefits: Strengthens the core muscles (abdomen) and improves balance both physically and mentally.

Precautions: Do not try this posture if you are pregnant or have lower back injuries or discomfort.

Boat Pose *(Navasana)*

Hold on to the back of the thighs as you lift the spine. Extend the arms out in line with the knees and feet and/or stretch the legs creating a "V" shape. Hold for 1 to 5 slow, deep breaths. Lift the belly towards the thighs. Relax the shoulders and jaw in this pose.

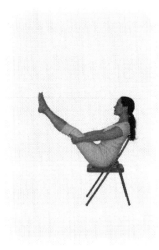

Hand Behind the Thighs

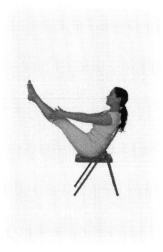

Arms and Legs Stretched

Benefits: Strengthens the core muscles (abdomen) and improves balance both physically and mentally.

Precautions: Do not try this posture if you are pregnant or have lower back injuries or discomfort.

Seated Archer Pose *(Akarna Dhanurasana)*

Make fists with your hands, keeping the thumbs up. Pull your right hand towards the right shoulder as you stretch the left hand out in the other direction, as if you were pulling a bow and arrow. Focus on the thumbnail of your left hand. Take 5 slow, deep breaths. Switch sides. Focus the eyes and the mind on your thumbnail. You can also visualize a goal in your life as you do this, imagining you are achieving your goal, as you keep a focus in your body and on the breath.

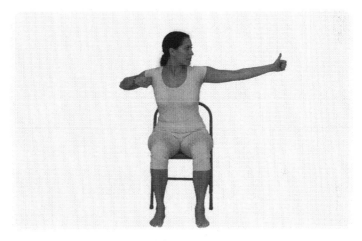

Archer Pose

Benefits: Improves focus and concentration. This pose strengthens the arms and opens the collarbone area (front of the chest) and shoulders. It gives strength to the mind and helps you visualize your goals clearly, with a sense of tranquility.

Inversions

Legs on the Chair Pose

Sit down on the floor with the side of your body facing the chair front. Lower yourself down to your elbows then onto your back, using your hands and arms to support you. Then bring the legs up on the chair. Place the hands about one foot from the hips with the palms facing up towards the sky. Keep the head centered over the spine. Close your eyes. Relax your body and mind. Hold the posture for 3 to 5 minutes or longer if you are comfortable. See the next page for how to come out of the posture safely and gently.

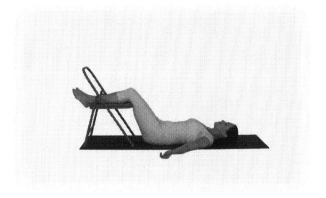

Legs on the Chair Pose

Benefits: Eases lower back pain, assists in circulation and relaxes the nervous system.

Precautions: For blood pressure issues and other medical concerns, lie flat on your back (if you are advised to not invert the legs).

How to Come Out of Legs on the Chair Pose

To come out of the posture safely and gently from Legs on the Chair Pose stretch one or both arms overhead.

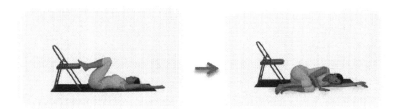

*Stretch one or both arms overhead. Roll to one side.
Rest the head on the outstretched arm and pause.*

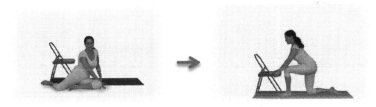

*Use your arms/hands to sit up and the legs to stand.
Use the chair base for support.*

Benefits: Eases lower back pain, assists in circulation and draining lymph from the lower legs and feet towards the heart.

Precautions: Check with your doctor for any medical concerns. If it is difficult or causes strain to lie on the floor, you can rest the feet up on a second chair and rest there. (See next page)

Legs on the Chair Pose Upright

Bring the legs up on a second chair in front of you. Place the hands on the thighs to rest or overhead for an active posture.

Resting Variation: If the hands are resting on the thighs, the palms can face up towards the sky or faced down if that is more comfortable. Keep the head centered over the spine. You can also place a pillow behind the lower back for support. Close the eyes. Relax your body and mind. Hold for 3 to 10 minutes.

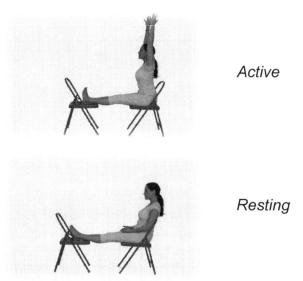

Active

Resting

Benefits: The inversions with chairs can have a similar benefit as full yoga inversions (turning the body upside down). It reverses the flow of blood and fluids from standing upright and stimulates the parasympathetic nervous system for calming the nervous system and calming the mind. This also helps reduce jet lag, insomnia and general feelings of stress and exhaustion (mental or physical).

Restorative Yoga Postures

Restorative Fish Pose *(Matsyasana)*

With props: You will need a yoga mat, towel or blanket.

Restorative: Roll up a blanket, towel or yoga mat. Place it behind you, running vertically along the spine. Rest back into the roll so that your back feels supported. Keep the head centered over the spine if the yoga mat does not support your head. Exhale, as you allow your shoulders to relax away from the ears and the tips of the shoulders towards the chair back. Hold for 1 to 5 minutes passively, letting go of all muscular tension or effort.

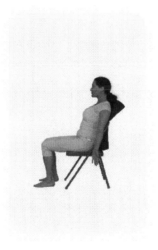

With Back Support

Benefits: Opens the upper back, relaxes the back, neck and shoulders, nervous system and the mind. It stimulates the parasympathetic nervous system for calming, restoring energy and healing. Allows the body to feel support, which may translate to feeling emotionally supported.

Supported Fish Pose Movements *(Matsyasana)*

With props: You will need a yoga mat, towel or blanket.

From the Restorative Fish Pose (see previous page) you can try some active arm variations as seen in the photos below. Breathe slowly as you lift the arms up overhead (or out to the sides). Exhale as you relax in the posture. Repeat these movements 3x.

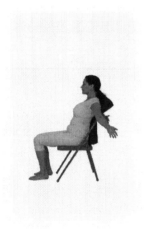

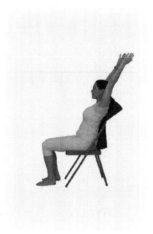

Fish With Support   *Active Arm Variations*

Benefits: Opens the upper back, relaxes the back, neck and shoulders.

Restorative Heart Openers

With props: You will need a yoga block, towel or blanket.

Restorative: Place the yoga block or tightly rolled blanket, towel or mat horizontally behind the shoulder blades (behind the heart area). Rest the back into the block so that your shoulders feel contact with the prop behind it, as in the photo on the next page. Exhale, as you allow your shoulders to relax away from the ears and gentle press the shoulder blades towards the block or rolled prop. Hold for 1 to 3 minutes, focusing on the heart area as you breathe.

Active: Breathe slowly as you lift the arms up overhead (or out to the sides). Exhale as you relax in the posture. Repeat these movements 1 to 5x.

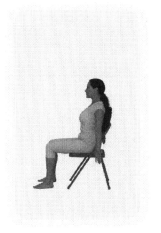 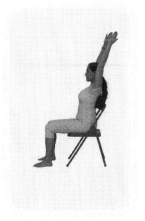

Restorative Heart Opener   *Arm Raises With Block*

Benefits: Opens the upper back and shoulders. Allows the heart area and upper back to open, which may translate to feeling emotionally more 'open hearted'. This posture is helpful after long hours at a computer, in a wheelchair or on an airplane where the upper back may tend to round forward.

YOGIC RELAXATION

Corpse Pose *(Savasana)*

Sitting in a chair, rest against the chair back. You can place pillows, blankets or a yoga mat behind your low back or along your spine or sit upright (instead of collapsing the low back or if there is any discomfort). The palms face up on the thighs or the arms can rest along side the chair with the palms facing forward or up. Relax and enjoy the benefits of your practice. Rest the muscles, the nerves and the mind.

If you are able to be on the floor, you can rest on your back, with the legs on the chair base. (See photo from Legs on the Chair Pose, which uses a second chair in front to elevate the legs). You can also rest in full Corpse Pose, which is done lying flat on the floor with the legs about 2 feet apart, the hands about a foot from the hips with the palms facing skyward. Keep the head centered.

Precautions: *For second and third trimester pregnancy adaptions, sit upright on the chair or rest on your side on the floor.

Final Relaxation

After each session of practicing the yoga exercises, postures and/or breath work, it is best to relax for 5 to15 minutes or more. Enjoy this time to integrate the physical postures and practice you just completed.

Chair Yoga Relaxation Postures

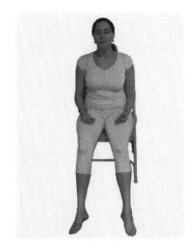

Corpse Pose

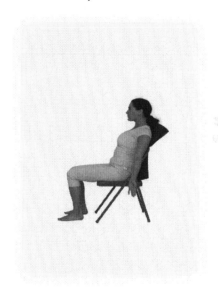

With Support

Relaxation Techniques

Tense and release each muscle in the body to feel the difference between tension and relaxation. Then you can practice "autosuggestion" by mentally repeating, "I relax my toes, my toes relax", as you bring awareness to the toes. Feel the toes relax from deep within. Then shift the awareness to the ankles as you repeat silently, "I relax my ankles, my ankles relax." Repeat with the knees, legs, low back, hips, middle back, upper back, stomach, digestive organs, heart, lungs, shoulders, arms, elbows, wrists, hands, fingers, neck, throat, jaw, eyes, scalp and ears (in this order). Rest in complete silence for 5 to 15 minutes or as needed. Ease out of the posture slowly and sit upright. Meditate on the breath for a few minutes.

Benefits: Final Relaxation in *Savasana* (Corpse Pose) relaxes the physical body, nervous system and the mind. This gives us time to integrate the physical exercises and breathing practices. It stimulates the parasympathetic nervous system for calming, restoring energy and healing. This is especially helpful when recovering from injuries, chronic illness or posttraumatic stress and is good in general for us all to do daily to ease the nerves from daily stress.

Closing Chants/Mantras/Prayers

You can repeat out loud or silently:
Om *shanti, shanti, shanti* or Om peace, peace, peace.

Add other mantras or other uplifting prayers or songs you may resonate with to bring feelings of joy and/or deep peace. Feel the peace of your true essence.

YOGA WORKS AT WORK

"Yoga works at work" is SunLight Chair Yoga's motto for offering yoga at the work place. You can do yoga at your desk at work or at home to avoid repetitive stress injuries; to ease neck, shoulder and back tension; to ease blurry vision syndrome from extensive computer use and to keep focused and refreshed during work or when you feel stress. You can do this without having to change into workout clothes or leaving your desk.

All of the exercises, postures breath work and meditations in this book can be done at work. Particularly good are the neck, shoulder and wrist exercises. However, all are equally beneficial to keep the body flexible and relaxed. Here is an example of a short work break you can take:

3 minute Shoulder and Neck Release sequence

- Take three slow, deep breaths. Feel yourself relax.

- Inhale as you shrug (slide) your shoulders up to the ears. Exhale as you drop and lower them. Repeat 3 to 6x. Imagine all of your tensions and worries leaving you with each exhalation.

- Inhale as you stretch your arms overhead. Exhale as you lower the arms. Repeat 3 to 6x.

- Rotate your wrists and ankles in circles. Repeat 5x in each direction.

Eagle Pose for Shoulder Tension *(Garudasana)*

Sit tall and relaxed with the head centered over the spine. Feel your feet on the floor. Relax your shoulders. Cross your right arm over the left as in the photo below. Cross the ankles or legs as well (optional). Bend the elbows. Lift the elbows up as you pull the shoulders down simultaneously. Enjoy 3 to 5x deep breaths. Switch sides.

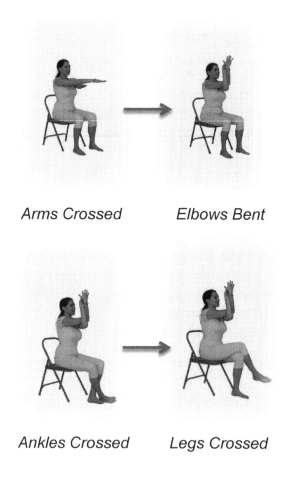

Arms Crossed   *Elbows Bent*

Ankles Crossed   *Legs Crossed*

Benefits: Releases tension in the upper back, neck and shoulders. Eases computer-related tensions and airplane travel-related tightness in the shoulders or from sitting long hours at a desk, in a chair or wheelchair.

Eagle Pose Variation

From Eagle Pose, bend forward, keeping the arms in the Eagle Pose position. Allow the shoulders and arms to relax and release into gravity.

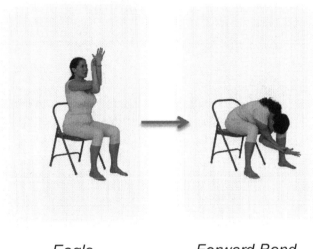

Eagle   *Forward Bend*

Benefits: Releases tension in the upper back, neck and shoulders. Eases computer-related tensions and airplane travel-related tightness in the shoulders or from sitting long hours at a desk, in a chair or wheelchair.

Cows Face Pose *(Gomukhasana)*

Sit tall and relaxed with the head centered over the spine. Feel your feet on the floor. Relax your shoulders.

Stretch your right arm to the right, with the thumb facing down and the palm facing the wall behind you. Rotate the arm bone until the thumb points to the back wall, or as far as you are comfortable. Reach the back of the palm to the touch the back.

Lift your left arm up by your ear, as in the photo below.

Bend your left elbow and try to reach the fingers towards each other. If the fingers touch, let them interlock. Otherwise use a strap or yoga belt like in the photo below.

If able, move the elbows towards the midline (center of head) so that the upper arm and the lower arm are moving towards the center of the spine. Rest your head back into your upper arm. Cross one ankle or leg over the other. Hold for 1 to 5 slow, deep breaths. Switch sides. (You can also do a forward bend in this posture.)

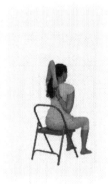

*See photos on the next page.

Getting Into the Cows Face Pose *(Gomukhasana)*

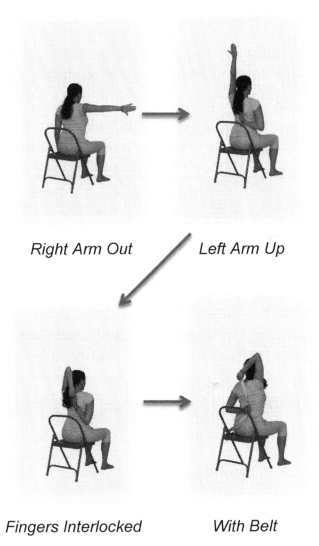

Right Arm Out   *Left Arm Up*

Fingers Interlocked   *With Belt*

Benefits: Releases tension in the upper back, neck and shoulders.

One-Minute Meditation for Stress Relief

Sit in a comfortable position with the spine tall but not tense. Feel your feet on the floor. Support the low back with a pillow if needed. Close your eyes. Bring yourself into the present moment. Become aware of your body and surroundings. Take a few deep sighs. Observe then regulate the breath with rhythmic, deep and slow breathing. Allow the mind to wander at first. Focus at the brow point (between the eyebrows), the navel or the heart center where the mind can rest. When the mind drifts, bring it back to the breath, which takes you back to the present moment.

Start with one minute a day for a week. Even if your mind isn't calm during the meditation, you will see the effects after daily practice. Increase this as time goes on to 3 minutes, then 5 minutes. You can do this at your desk in a chair, or in the mornings or evenings in a quiet place at home. Be regular in your 1 to 5 minute meditation practice for the best results.

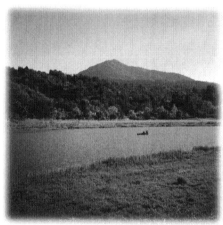

Observe and allow the thought waves to settle.

Eye Exercises *(Netra Vyayam)*

Here are some old, traditional yoga exercises for the eyes, specifically helpful in the modern era to ease computer-related vision issues, including getting dry and irritated or blurry eyes from long hours looking at the computer screen.

Sit tall in the chair, keeping the breath relaxed and rhythmic. Try not to move the head during the eye exercises.

- Up and down: Roll the eyes up and down. Repeat 5x.

- Side to side: Roll the eyes right to left, 5x. (See photo)

- Diagonals: Roll the eyes to the upper right corner, then to the lower left. Repeat 5x. Switch directions. Roll the eyes to the upper left corner, then to the lower right corner.

- Circles: Roll the eyes in circles clockwise. Try to even out the movement as best you can. Repeat 3 to 5x. Reverse the direction, circling the eyes counterclockwise.

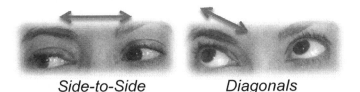

Side-to-Side   *Diagonals*

Benefits: Eases dryness or blurry vision. This helps when looking at a computer screen for long periods of time, increases concentration and is said to improve the eyesight.

BREATHING EXERCISES

Yoga breathing exercises, called pranayama, can be done at the beginning of the yoga session, at the end or by themselves. There are multiple benefits. Prana in Sanskrit is the "vital life force," that which gives us breath and life. Controlling the breath with these exercises is a start to learn how to control the vital life force, that which gives us energy and sustains us. With daily practice the benefits are infinite, including bringing more oxygen to the blood and cells of the body, purifying the nerves and calming the mind.

Breathing Exercises *(Pranayama)*

To begin, sit tall in a chair as best you can without any strain. Have the feet hip-width apart, with the feet on the floor. (If you are in wheelchair, modify as needed.) Sit away from the chair back and upright for Alternate Nostril Breath. Slow Deep Breathing and Three-Part Breath (Full Yogic Breath) can also be done lying down if needed. Sitting upright creates a feeling of centering the mind and creating alertness. At the end of the yoga exercises, or before relaxation, this can be done in a relaxation pose or lying down for relaxation effects.

Precautions: Take slow, deep breaths if the breathing techniques cause you discomfort or dizziness. Stop the exercise and rest. Try it again when you are ready. Only continue if you are comfortable and feel at ease. All of the breathing exercises in this book are safe for prenatal yoga (all trimesters).

"Breath is central to Yoga because breath is central to life...and Yoga is about life"
-T Krishnamacharya

Slow Deep Breathing

Sit tall in your chair with your eyes closed (or open if needed). You can also do this from any of the yoga postures in the book, including Legs on the Chair Pose and Relaxation Pose.

Take slow, deep, rhythmic breaths. Inhale and exhale through the nose (if able). Inhale for 3 counts. Exhale for 3 counts. While you count, you can mentally add an "Aum (OM)" mantra in between the numbers. (Ex: Om 1, Om 2, etc.) There should be no strain. The shoulders, face and throat remain relaxed. If comfortable, you can increase the breath to 4 counts as you inhale, and 4 counts as you exhale.

This breath type can be done during all yoga postures *(asanas)* too. This is good to do throughout the day, anywhere or anytime, especially in moments when you feel overwhelmed, anxious, angry or stressed out. Be aware of the breath as it connects to the body. Soon your emotions and mind will follow the breath for a deep sense of calm and inner peace.

Benefits: Centers the mind, reduces anxiety, stimulates the parasympathetic nervous system for calming, helps regulate sleep and digestive imbalances. This is a simple and effective 'yogic tool' that can be done anywhere without anyone even knowing you are practicing yoga!

Three-Part (Full Yogic) Breath

- Bring the hands to the navel area (belly) as in the photo below.

- Inhale into the belly (push your hands out with the belly as you inhale, expanding the lower belly like a balloon, with no strain.) Exhale and relax. Inhale and exhale for 3 counts each.

- Bring one hand to upper chest. Keep the other hand on the lower abdomen.

- Inhale into the lower abdomen, then the middle torso, then the upper chest in 3 parts. Exhale in reverse, in 3 counts.

When you feel comfortable with the breath, you can relax the hands on the thighs and continue. Repeat 3-10 rounds. Note: You can mentally repeat, "OM 1, OM 2, OM 3", as you count, adding the mantra OM between each number.

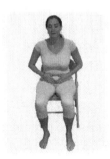

Hands on Abdomen

Benefits: Relaxes the stomach, calms and centers the mind, stimulates the parasympathetic nervous system. You can do this anywhere and anytime you feel anxious or stressed.

Alternate Nostril Breath

Place the right hand in Vishnu Mudra (index and middle finger in towards the palm). (See photo below) Use the thumb to close the right nostril and the ring finger to close the left nostril, alternating sides. If you are more comfortable or as needed, you can do this with the palm flat and the fingers stretched up. Switch from the index finger to close the left nostril and the ring finger to close the right nostril. (See photos below)

Inhale through the left nostril for 4 counts (block the right nostril with the thumb). Exhale through the right nostril for 8 counts, using the hand position above to close and release the alternating nostrils. Inhale through the right nostril for 4 counts and exhale through the left nostril for 8 counts. Repeat 3 to 12 rounds. The focus is on the third eye (between the eyebrows), with the eyes closed during this exercise. Keep the spine tall yet relaxed.

Return to slow, deep breathing at any point and rest the arm if needed. Pranayama works best when the body is relaxed.

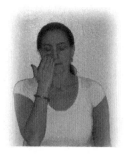
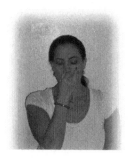

Palm Flat   *Vishnu Mudra*

Alternate Nostril Breath Benefits

Benefits: Balances the right and left-brain and the energies of the body, calms for the nervous system and mind, improves sleep and concentration abilities, regulates the digestive functions by stimulating the relaxation response and turns the focus inward. This is also a useful preparation for meditation.

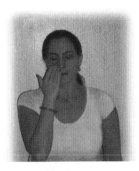
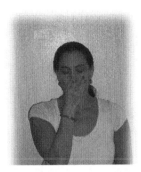

Palm Flat   *Vishnu Mudra*

Selected Yoga Sutras (from Patanjali)

Sutra 1.2 (Sanskrit): *yogascittavrittinirodhah*

Translation: Yoga is the ability to focus the mind towards one point or object and sustain focus in that direction without distraction. Or, Yoga is the stopping of the mind fluctuations.

Sutra 1.14 (Sanskrit) *sa tu dirghakala nairantarya satkara asevitah drdhabhumih*

Translation: Consistent, alert practice with enthusiasm is the firm foundation for stopping the mind fluctuations.

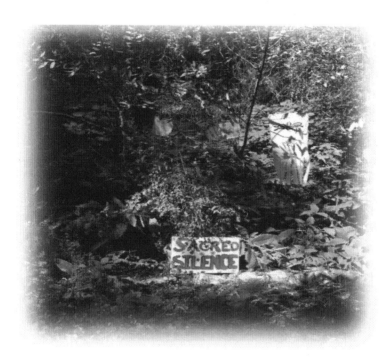

MEDITATION

Meditation is a time-tested tool for stress reduction and increasing inner peace. It is calming for the mind, brings clarity and increases intuition and our ability to concentrate. In Sanskrit, meditation or dhyana is the ability to hold the focus of the mind on one object without distraction until you are absorbed in the focal point, merging with that point of focus. Focusing on a candle (tratak, or "eye gazing"), a sound, or mantra or breath are some common focal points. Try to pick something calming or uplifting for the mind.

You can gain many health benefits. For instance, meditation has been studied and proven to reduce heart disease. However, studying it alone does not give you the full benefit. It only works when you do it!

Thinking of meditation, intending to practice and learning its philosophy are helpful but alone will not give you the fruits of the practice. When meditation is done with consistent practice, regardless of how busy the mind is, we can access a deep well of joy and peace. Often my yoga students say that they or their minds need to meditate. When we sit still, regardless of the reasons why we think we can't, that act of discipline teaches us again and again that we are the masters of our own minds and more than our thoughts alone. Who is the silent witness and knower of all your thoughts? Let's check it out, in one short but sweet minute.

How to Meditate

Find a quiet place. Sit in a comfortable position with your spine tall but not tense. In a chair, you can sit tall with the feet on the floor. Support the lower back with a pillow if needed. Close your eyes. Bring yourself into the present moment. Become aware of your body and its surroundings. Take a few deep sighs. Inhale through the nose. Exhale through the mouth or nose. Start to regulate the breath. Begin slow, rhythmic, deep breathing. Start to observe the breath. Allow the mind to wander at first. It may jump around, but will eventually become quiet. Focus on a point between the eyebrows or the heart area where the mind can rest. When the mind drifts, bring it back to the moment and become aware of the breath. Start with one minute a day. Increase the meditation period gradually over time. Practice, practice, practice!

Be patient with yourself. This takes time to develop. However, the benefits are worth it! If you meditate daily, you will be able to face life with more peace and inner strength, having an anchor within yourself through difficult times. Even if the mind does not seem calm and thoughts are endless, you can still receive the benefits and feel more centered throughout your day. Consistent practice is key.

"Get up now. This is Brahmamuhurta (Auspicious Early Morning Time). Everywhere is silence. Nature herself is at peace. Now you can retire peacefully into the inner chambers of your heart."Sivananda

MANTRAS AND CHANTING

Yoga is commonly thought of as physical exercises and breathing techniques, perhaps with some relaxation. However, that is part of Hatha Yoga. There are also other branches of yoga that do not require any physical abilities or mobility.

The Sivananda Yoga lineage summarizes the paths of yoga in this way: "There are four main paths of Yoga - Karma Yoga, Bhakti Yoga, Raja Yoga and Jnana Yoga. Each is suited to a different temperament or approach to life…. Swami Sivananda recognized that every Yogi, or human being for that matter, possesses and identifies with each of these elements: Intellect, heart, body and mind. He therefore advocated that everyone practice certain techniques from each path. This came to be known as the Yoga of Synthesis. He also taught that, in accordance with individual temperament and taste, one can emphasize the practice of certain Yogas over others." www.sivananda.org

Mantras and chanting are apart of Bhakti Yoga, which is the yogic path of devotion. This can be done at the end of the yoga session or on its own. Feel the joy in your heart and soul and you chant and sing with devotion. Chanting is not like singing or performing. Your voice does not have to be "good" or you do not have to feel it is "good" to chant and feel the inner joy it brings. If you are new to chanting and prefer to chant silently, you can still feel and reap the benefits. Although you can chant in any language, the Sanskrit language is said to have a spiritual resonance, as it was spoken from the gurus from thousands of years ago and carried through the ages.

Mantras

AUM (OM)

Inhale. As you exhale, chant AUM (OM). Feel as if you are chanting from deep within the navel center, letting the sound current (wave) rise up to the third eye point (point between the eyebrows). Imagine that every cell of your body is being healed by the sacred primordial sound of the universe: AUM.

Universal prayer for the welfare of all beings
Lokha, Samasta Sukino, Bhavantu (Repeat 3x)

Aum (Om). Shanti, Shanti, Shanti-e

Translation: May all beings in all worlds be blessed with freedom, health and happiness. Om, we invoke the Divine Primordial Source Energy to fill us with: Peace to our bodies, Peace in our minds, Peace to all souls.

Ancient prayer for knowing our inner, eternal and true Self:

Asato Ma Sat Gamaya
Lead us from the unreal to the real.
Tamasoma Jyotir Gamaya
Lead us from darkness to light.
Mrityor Maamritam Gamaya
Lead us from fear of death/anxiety,
To knowledge of our eternal soul.
Aum. Shanti, Shanti, Shanti-e
Peace. Peace. Peace.

ShalOM, ShalOM, ShalOM Peace Peace Peace
(This is not a traditional yoga mantra, but Hebrew.)

Kirtan Kriya for Memory Improvement

Yogi Bhajan, who brought Kundalini Yoga to the west, taught Kirtan Kriya. It is a combination of mantras and mudras (chants and hand postures). The mantras are from the Gurmukhi script from India. The other chants in the book and the names of the yoga postures are in the Sanskrit language, also from India.

The following description of how to do this exercise (or meditation) is written by the Alzheimer's Research & Prevention Foundation. (See the reference section for more details on how their evidence-based study showed that this Kirtan Kriya improved memory in patients suffering from mild cognitive impairment (MCI) and early Alzheimer's.)

The Alzheimer's Research & Prevention Foundation has assembled this information on the Kirtan Kriya singing exercise for medical professionals, the public, caregivers, the media and anyone interested in improving brain function and slowing memory loss.

The Kirtan Kriya exercise uses the primal sounds and is meant to be practiced for greater attention, concentration, focus, improved short-term memory and better mood. The primal sounds consist of: Saa – means Birth or Infinity, Taa – means Life, Naa – means Death or Transformation, Maa – means Rebirth.

The sounds are chanted repeatedly and in order (i.e., Saa Taa Naa Maa). You can start with 3 minutes until you are familiar with the technique, using the time ratio of 30 s:30 s:60 s:30 s:30 s and then building up to a full 12 minutes.

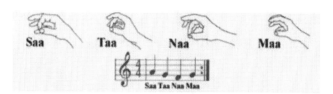

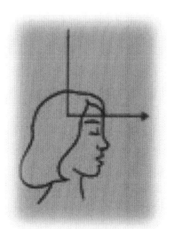

L Form Visualization

Kirtan Kriya Singing Exercise Instructions

If you would like to practice the Kirtan Kriya singing exercise, here are the basic steps:

1. Repeat the Saa Taa Naa Maa sounds (or mantra) while sitting with your spine straight. If possible, your focus of concentration is the L form (see illustration on the left), with your eyes are closed. With each syllable, imagine the sound flowing in through the top of your head and out the middle of your forehead (your third eye point, as in the illustration on the left).

2. For 2 minutes, sing in your normal voice.

3. For the next 2 minutes, sing in a whisper.

4. For the next 4 minutes, say the sound silently to yourself.

5. Then reverse the order, whispering for 2 minutes, and then out loud for 2 minutes, for a total of 12 minutes.

6. To come out of the exercise, inhale very deeply, stretch your hands above your head, and then bring them down slowly in a sweeping motion as you exhale.

The finger positions are very important in this kriya:

• On Saa, touch the index fingers of each hand to your thumbs.
• On Taa, touch your middle fingers to your thumbs.
• On Naa, touch your ring fingers to your thumbs.
• On Maa, touch your little fingers to your thumbs.

YOGIC DIET

Yoga exercises, breathing practices, relaxation, meditation and mantras are all helpful for a more balanced and healthy body and a peaceful mind. What we put into our bodies is just as important as the other aspects of the yoga lifestyle. Maybe even more so because of the fact that we eat every day!

Shifting to or keeping a vegetarian diet to help create a healthier body and a more peaceful mind can be a very simple process. Just as we brush our teeth and shower to keep our body clean, often without much thought, so we can eat foods that keep us clean and nourish us on the inside as well, all while not harming ourselves, the environment or animals in the process.

Ahimsa (nonviolence) is the first principle in the philosophy of yoga, establishing a base to keep the physical body healthy and the mind less agitated. Most of the yoga masters teach that it is difficult to control your mind when you are eating meat (there are scientific reasons for this, including the adrenalin and hormones associated with the way the animals are raised and slaughtered, among others). All of the myths and debates about why one needs meat have been disproven in this modern age, and in fact it has been shown that vegetarian diet is healthier.

Yogic diet is a lacto-ovo vegetarian diet, one in which vegetables, fruits, nuts, grains and dairy are eaten in balance to create optimal health and vitality.

With the proper balance of the protein and nutrients your body needs, you can feel more energy and vitality. Keeping it simple, not eating too much or too little protein and balancing our meals with vegetables, grains and protein, while making it appealing to yourself, creates a diet that is "easeful, useful, and peaceful", as Swami Sachidananda used to say that yoga (and life) should be.

It seems many are now "going green" by recycling more and being more mindful of eating organic foods and such. In fact, the most support one can offer Mother Earth is to eat less or no meat. "You save more water by not eating a pound of meat than you do by not showering for six months!" as calculated by PETA.

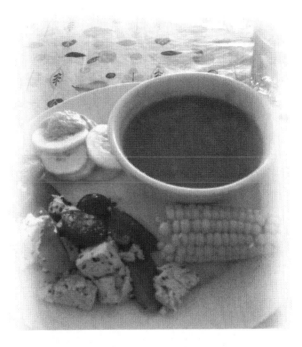

A Well Balanced Vegetarian Meal

Here is more on the topic of yogic diet and the environment:

"Green Plate Special," Save the Earth in a Bite

"Nothing will benefit human health and increase the chances of survival of life on earth as much as the evolution to a vegetarian diet." - Albert Einstein

Many people are "going green" to save resources and sustain the planet. Shifting to a plant-based diet supports your personal health as well as the health of our Mother Earth. As yogis, there is a long tradition of living in harmony with the earth and its inhabitants.

Ahimsa is the Sanskrit term for "nonviolence." Living as a yogi, it makes sense to shift to a vegetarian lifestyle. This way of being embraces the concept of not harming ourselves, our bodies, the earth we live on or the animals, both wild and domesticated. In addition to feeling more energy, vitality and lightness of the body when practicing yoga, you help "green" the earth by reducing or abstaining from eating meat—one bite at a time!

A vegetarian diet helps heal the planet by conserving fossil fuels- it takes significantly more energy to produce meat products than to grow plant foods. We are all learning how critical it is to reduce our carbon "footprint." We help the planet when we buy organic and locally grown produce as well, since we reduce transportation impacts and help with soil conservation.

There are so many reasons why a plant-based diet is an effective and easy way to "go green"-by eating in a healthy way for yourself and the planet. You will improve your personal health, support your yoga practice and do your part to heal the planet every time you sit down to a meal. Make a New Year's resolution to learn more about your connection to the food you eat. "Go green" to get healthier and bless the earth in 2012. www.yogamint.com Jan. 2012

Enjoy this recipe for its protein with steamed greens and/or salad for a healthy and simple meal. Note: You can also shave some fresh ginger to put on top before baking, and if you are vegan, substitute the butter with oil to coat the pan and put tamari on top of the tofu.

This is from the Sivananda Yoga Cookbook:

BAKED TOFU RECIPE

Serves 4

Ingredients:

1lb. tofu
Block butter
Tamari
Good-tasting yeast

Instructions:

Slice the tofu into 10 to 12 slices. Melt butter in a saucepan and add tamari for flavor. Layer the tofu in a cookie sheet or large pan and then pour the butter-tamari mixture over it. Sprinkle some yeast on top of the tofu, and bake in the oven at 375 degrees Fahrenheit for 20 minutes or until the tofu is lightly roasted and crispy.

Additional Vegetarian Recipes

Another recipe from the Sivananda Yoga Cookbook and ashrams:

Sunflower Seed Salad Dressing

This is the most popular salad dressing in the Sivananda Yoga ashrams worldwide. Try some on your leafy greens!

Blend 1 C oil, 1/2 C tamari, 1/2 C lemon juice and 1 to 2 C sunflower seeds until you get a smooth and creamy consistency. If the consistency is too thick, add some water; if too thin, add more sunflower seeds. To this mixture, you can add any herb or spice you prefer. Taste and adjust. Makes 4-5 cups.

STACIE'S KALE CHIP RECIPE

For a healthy snack at home or work, try kale chips. This is a healthy alternative to potato chips.

Preheat the oven to 360-370 degrees. Put olive oil in a pan. Bake small pieces of kale broken up (or cut up) at 370 degrees Fahrenheit, with olive oil lightly sprinkled on before baking. Add some salt.

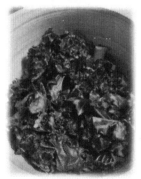

Kale Chips

SUNLIGHT CHAIR YOGA ARTICLES

"Learning Yoga at 82" KQED Radio (NPR) 2012

Joseph Levine: In our first-person series "What's Your Story?", Californians talk about health in their lives and communities. One of the more unlikely yogis you'll meet on the mat is 82-year-old Joseph Levine, who lives in a retirement community in Marin County.

"We have stereotypes, and whenever I would see a magazine or there would a little short about India on television. You would see these fellas, naked with ashes on their heads with legs around their head. And I always knew I couldn't do that.

"Frankly when I began, I didn't know whether I'd be able to do it. I looked around at these old ladies and I said, 'By God I can't put shame to my sex, I've got to make the effort!' And I found it came on comparatively easily. Because it's very gentle very gentle.

"I'm always grateful that I come out of it alive, and that I can keep up. And slowly I'm building up my courage to wrap. To wrap one foot around another and not hold on to the chair for dear life is progress for me.

"My voice is a little bit gravely now. And I'm actually attending speech therapy session and I can't bring the volume up to speak [loud.] But it doesn't affect my singing. It's like it comes from a different place, and I reach down and sing. But talking is harder. So I guess we have bodies within bodies, and they know what they can do given the opportunity.

"I'm drawing on resources within me that I don't produce outside of this setting. But here, it's kinda a warm up, and we don't get to chanting until all of the switches on the dashboard are on as it were. And there's an element of joy, when I can bring my voice and reach. I fly. It's a high. And when I'm through with the entire session there's a certain peacefulness. Of course lunch is coming, that always thrills me."

"Yoga for Seniors" CBS Ch. 4 Health Watch 2011

MIAMI BEACH – Keeping seniors active can be key to both their mental and physical health. There's now a new way for seniors to stay active thanks to a special kind of Yoga class geared specifically for seniors.

The moves are fluid and require grace and poise, but for the poses we are writing about, standing is not required. Stacie Dooreck is a yoga Instructor that is breathing new life into South Florida seniors. She owns SunLight Yoga in South Florida. "If you are in a chair and your hips hurt or your knees hurt, you can do the arm movement in a yoga pose," said Stacie Dooreck.

The point is to keep the muscles active, but how does that happen sitting down? "Sitting in a chair, you get a similar effect for the flow of energy and circulation," Dooreck said to CBS4's Jorge Estevez at the Miami Beach Senior Center, where the seniors were learning Yoga.

The practice seemed to work. "I learned a lot of things today. This exercise with the hands," Angelina Rodriguez said after class. The practice is not only good for their bodies, but also their minds. "You have to continue moving until you go the grave," joked Jose Soler who also took the class. "You are meeting people to socialize with you have something to look forward to, so it affects you both emotionally and physically," said Joyce Kagan, Director of the Jewish Community services who holds the classes in her center. Yoga can be a great exercise for seniors, but regardless of what kind of movement you want to do, the goal is to stay active.

"Road Trip Yoga" Marin Magazine 2013

Heading out of town this weekend? We've got the solution to road trip / plane ride blahs! Road Trip Yoga is a collection for great chair poses by Stacie Dooreck of Larkspur, California from her book, *SunLight Chair Yoga*. These simple moves can help prevent stiffness and increase blood flow (keep your mind and body happy!) without leaving your seat.

Centering Sit in a comfortable position with the spine tall yet relaxed. Take a few deep, sighing breaths. Inhale and exhale for three counts each, five times.

Wrist and Ankle Rotations Rotate the wrists, then the ankles- five times each.

Neck Rolls Slowly make a circle with your nose five times in each direction, clockwise and counterclockwise. Inhale when facing upward and exhale when looking down. Keep shoulders relaxed.

Alternate Leg Lifts Inhale as you raise your lower leg from a bent knee, and exhale as you bring it back down. Switch sides. Repeat up to five times.

Alternate Arm Lifts Inhale as you lift your right arm. Exhale as you lower the arm. Switch sides. Repeat five times each.

Combine Arm and Leg Lifts Inhale as you lift the right arm and left leg together. Exhale as you lower them. Switch. Make diagonal movements. Keep the spine tall.

Mountain Pose Sit tall in a chair. Lift from the base of your spine through the crown of your head. Feel the strength of the back muscles and the sides of your body lifting. Keep feet on the floor.

Side Stretch (Crescent Moon) Inhale, sitting tall, as you lengthen the spine skyward. Exhale, facing forward, as you lean gently to the right, placing your right hand by your right hip or letting it hang beside the chair, and raising your left hand to extend it over the left ear. Switch sides. Repeat three times on each side.

Cat to Cobra Pose/Spinal Flex Inhale to Cobra — lift your chest and heart as your hands slide to your hips along the thighs. Bring the elbows toward each other. Exhale to Cat — move your belly toward your spine as you round your back with arms stretched straight and hands on knees. Repeat up to 10 times.

Spinal Twist Place feet on the floor, hip-width apart. Inhale as you sit tall. Lengthen the spine skyward. Exhale and twist gently to the right, placing your right hand behind you or on the side of the chair and your left hand on or near the right knee. Switch sides. Only twist as far as is comfortable, with no strain. You can repeat this posture once on each side.

Final Relaxation Rest your back against the chair with your legs one to two feet apart. Allow the legs to roll outward. Relax your arms with palms facing the sky, resting on your thighs. Observe the breath and body; relax for five to 10 minutes. Quiet the spirit and calm the mind. Slowly move your hands and feet to come out of the position and sit tall.

REFERENCES

1- Light on Yoga by BKS Iyengar lists in great detail the benefits of over 500 yoga postures. Although this book has yoga postures that are different (because they are adapted in chairs), many of the benefits are similar. For example, the upper body benefits to Warrior Posture would be the same as the standing version. Light on Yoga says, "The chest is fully expanding and it helps deep breathing, relieves stiffness in the shoulders and back and cures stiffness in the neck."

2- Evidence-based studies for fall prevention are discussed at www.projectenhance.org. Many of the exercises studied and evidence-based research proved that doing these exercises does prevent falls among seniors and those with balance challenges other related issues. Some of these yoga postures, although not studied in the yoga format (moving with breath), are similar to or the same as the exercises studied, utilizing the same muscles needed for strength and stability.

3- Yoga Sutras in more detail, with translations, are in The Heart of Yoga by TKV Desikachar and The Yoga Sutras of Patanjali by Swami Sachidanana.

4- An evidence-based study of yoga mantras and mudras (hand postures) to improve memory in patients suffering from Mild Cognitive Impairment (MCI) and early Alzheimer's was done by Dr. Dharma Singh Khalsa, M.D., Alzheimer's Research and Prevention Foundation in AZ: www.alzheimersprevention.org.

5- www.yogajournal.com on yoga postures.

RECOMMENDED BOOKS & APP

The Sivananda Companion to Meditation:
How to Master the Mind by the Sivananda Yoga Centers

The Sivananda Companion to Yoga by the Sivananda Yoga Centers

The Yoga Cookbook by the Sivananda Yoga Centers:

Light on Yoga by BKS Iyengar

The Heart of Yoga by TKV Desikachar

The Yoga Sutras of Patanjali by Swami Sachidanana

Books and DVD's by Lilias Folan

Ahimsa: nonviolent eating: recipes and chair yoga for digestion http://ahimsa.sunlightchairyoga.com

SunLight Yoga Chair Yoga videos and app (free):
www.sunlightchairyoga.com

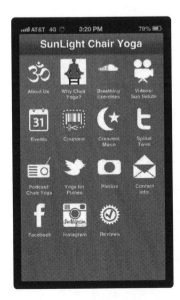

ABOUT THE AUTHOR

Stacie Dooreck (Saraswati) was born and raised a vegetarian and taken to yoga ashrams since birth. Stacie began teaching yoga in 1995 (Sivananda Certified) and since became certified to teach prenatal yoga, Gentle Integral Yoga and Kundalini Yoga as taught by Yogi Bhajan. In addition, Stacie trained at the advanced studies program at the Iyengar Institute of San Francisco and continues to study with the masters.

After needing to adapt her own yoga practice during an illness and receiving its healing benefits, Stacie loves to share the joy and benefits of yoga with others. Stacie created and leads the SunLight Chair Yoga teacher trainings in NY, NM, CA, FL and in the Bahamas.

Stacie is also the author of Ahimsa: nonviolent eating book and ebook (http://ahimsa.sunlightchairyoga.com) and wrote a 150 page manual for the SunLight Chair Yoga Teacher Trainings. Since 2005 Stacie writes a monthly *SunLight Yogatips* eletter and writes articles for magazines and websites.

Contact Information:

For SunLight Chair Yoga teacher trainings information or to host a SunLight Chair Yoga teacher training in your area, contact:

Email: info@sunlightyoga.com
www.facebook.com/yogainchairs
www.twitter/yogainchairs
www.sunlightchairyoga.com

ORDERING BOOKS

To order books for individuals or wholesale, or to donate a copy to your local library or assisted living home:

Email: info@sunlightyoga.com
Website: www.sunlightchairyoga.com

Tel: 415-68-YOGA-U (415-689-6428)

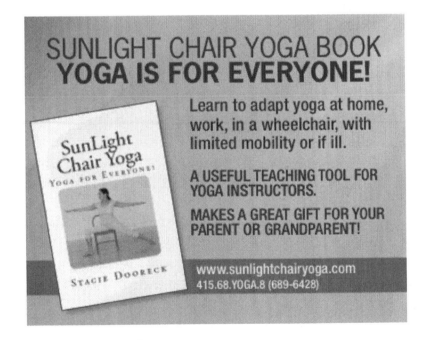